CONTENTS

Guidelines for
Antithrombotic Therapy
Eighth Edition

Jack Hirsh
CM, MD, FRCP(C), FRACP, FRSC, DSc

Professor Emeritus of Medicine
McMaster University
Director Emeritus
Henderson Research Centre
Hamilton, Ontario

2009
PEOPLE'S MEDICAL PUBLISHING HOUSE
Shelton, Connecticut

People's Medical Publishing House
2 Enterprise Drive, Suite 509
Shelton, CT 06484
Tel: 203-402-0646
Fax: 203-402-0854
E-mail: info@pmph-usa.com

PEOPLE'S MEDICAL PUBLISHING HOUSE

08 09 10 11 12/BMC/9 8 7 6 5 4 3 2

ISBN 978-1-60795-009-7
Printed in Canada by Ball Media Corporation
Typesetter: Norm Reid

Sales and Distribution

Canada
McGraw-Hill Ryerson Education
Customer Care
300 Water St
Whitby, Ontario L1N 9B6
Canada
Tel: 1-800-565-5758
Fax: 1-800-463-5885
www.mcgrawhill.ca

Foreign Rights
John Scott & Company
International Publisher's Agency
P.O. Box 878
Kimberton, PA 19442
USA
Tel: 610-827-1640
Fax: 610-827-1671

Japan
United Publishers Services Limited
1-32-5 Higashi-Shinagawa
Shinagawa-ku, Tokyo 140-0002
Japan
Tel: 03-5479-7251
Fax: 03-5479-7307
Email: kakimoto@ups.co.jp

United Kingdom, Europe,
Middle East, Africa
McGraw Hill Education
Shoppenhangers Road
Maidenhead
Berkshire, SL6 2QL
England
Tel: 44-0-1628-502500
Fax: 44-0-1628-635895
www.mcgraw-hill.co.uk

Singapore, Thailand, Philippines,
Indonesia, Vietnam, Pacific Rim, Korea
McGraw-Hill Education
60 Tuas Basin Link
Singapore 638775
Tel: 65-6863-1580
Fax: 65-6862-3354
www.mcgraw-hill.com.sg

Australia, New Zealand
Elsevier Australia
Tower 1, 475 Victoria Avenue
Chatswood NSW 2067
Australia
Tel: 0-9422-8553
Fax: 0-9422-8562
www.elsevier.com.au

Brazil
Tecmedd Importadora e
Distribuidora
de Livros Ltda.
Avenida Maurilio Biagi 2850
City Ribeirao, Rebeirao, Preto SP
Brazil
CEP: 14021-000
Tel: 0800-992236
Fax: 16-3993-9000
Email: tecmedd@tecmedd.com.br

India, Bangladesh, Pakistan,
Sri Lanka, Malaysia
CBS Publishers
4819/X1 Prahlad Street 24
Ansari Road, Darya, New Delhi-110002
India
Tel: 91-11-23266861/67
Fax: 91-11-23266818
Email:cbspubs@vsnl.com

People's Republic of China
PMPH
Bldg 3, 3rd District
Fangqunyuan, Fangzhuang
Beijing 100078
P.R. China
Tel: 8610-67653342
Fax: 8610-67691034
www.pmph.com

INTRODUCTION

In June 2008, the American College of Chest Physicians (ACCP) published the proceedings of the Eighth ACCP Conference on Antithrombotic and Thrombolytic Therapy: Evidence-Based Guidelines. The
proceedings of the ACCP Consensus Conference provide an extensive
critical review of the literature related to management of thromboembolic
disorders. We have added a chapter addressing the management of patients
who are treated with anticoagulants or antiplatelet drugs and who require
bridging therapy because of an intercurrent invasive procedure.

Since the first publication of the guidelines in 1986, the number of
antithrombotic agents available to the clinician has quadrupled, and the
rigor with which they are evaluated has improved dramatically. High-
quality studies in most fields have resulted in new and strong evidence-
based recommendations. There remains, however, a lack of randomized
trials in pediatric thrombosis, thrombosis in pregnancy, and thrombosis in
valvular heart disease.

The numbers of participants from outside North America has continued to increase, reflecting the widespread use of these guidelines
internationally.

Changes continue to be introduced to strengthen the methodology
used for the literature search. The search process is now more comprehen-
sive, transparent, and explicit. The authors provided the clinically relevant
questions, and the literature searches were conducted by a recognized evidence-based center at McMaster University.

The organization of the chapters has also been improved. In each chapter, the clinical question under consideration, the clinical trials evaluating
the evidence, and the recommendations are linked by a numbering scheme
common to these three items. This allows the reader to quickly identify the
underlying question associated with each recommendation as well as the
relevant evidence. The grading system in this edition of the ACCP guidelines now reflects the system adopted for all ACCP guidelines, and is similar to the Grades of Recommendation, Assessment, Development and
Evaluation (GRADE) system, which is being widely adopted by many
guideline groups.

This short monograph, which is an update of the 1992, 1995, 1998,
2001, and 2004 publications, provides a summary of the 2008 ACCP
recommendations, together with a brief review of the background data
on which the recommendations are based. Important clinical trials that
have been published after the last edition are described in more detail
than older trials. In order to keep the document short, no attempt is
made to provide detailed supporting evidence for the recommendations,

which can be obtained by referring to the proceeding of the Eighth ACCP Conference on Antithrombotic and Thrombolytic Therapy: Evidence-Based Guidelines.

1 GRADES OF RECOMMENDATION FOR ANTITHROMBOTIC AGENTS

The ACCP revised its system for grading recommendations used in evidence-based guidelines. This new grading system, although similar to the system used in past publications, was modified to conform with a grading scheme developed by the GRADE Working Group, which assesses the quality of evidence and strength of recommendations. This new grading system is being adopted by an increasing number of other organizations, including UpToDate, the American College of Physicians, the American Thoracic Society, and the World Health Organization.

The strength of any recommendation depends on two factors: the trade-off between benefits, risks, burden, and cost, and the level of confidence in estimates of those benefits and risks. As before, if guidelines developers are very certain that benefits do, or do not, outweigh risks, burden, and costs, they will make a strong recommendation—designated as **Grade 1**. If they are less certain of the magnitude of the benefits and risks, burden, and costs, they make a weaker **Grade 2** recommendation. Support for these recommendations may come from high-quality, moderate-quality, or low-quality evidence—labeled, respectively **A, B, and C**. The terms "we *recommend*" are used for strong recommendations **(grades 1A, 1B, 1C)** and "we *suggest*" for weaker recommendations **(grades 2A, 2B, 2C)**.

HOW METHODOLOGIC QUALITY CONTRIBUTES TO GRADES OF RECOMMENDATION

The highest quality evidence comes from one or more well-designed and well-executed randomized controlled trials (RCTs) yielding consistent and directly applicable results. High-quality evidence can also come from well-done observational studies yielding very large effects. *Moderate-quality evidence* comes from RCTs with important limitations and well-done observational studies yielding large effects. *Low-quality evidence* comes from well-done observational studies yielding modest effects or from RCTs with very serious limitations.

INTERPRETING THE RECOMMENDATIONS

In general, anything other than a **1A** recommendation indicates that the chapter authors acknowledge that other interpretations of the evidence, and other clinical policies, may be reasonable and appropriate. Even **Grade 1A** recommendations will not apply to all circumstances and all patients and may be influenced by the availability of resources and by patient preferences.

2 PARENTERAL ANTICOAGULANTS

The parenteral anticoagulants in current use can be divided into indirect anticoagulants, whose activity is mediated by plasma cofactors, and direct anticoagulants that do not require plasma cofactors to express their activity. The indirect parenteral anticoagulants in current use are heparin, low-molecular-weight heparin (LMWH), fondaparinux, and danaparoid. These drugs have little or no intrinsic anticoagulant activity, and exert their anti-coagulant activity by activating antithrombin (AT), an endogenous inhibitor of various activated clotting factors. The parenteral direct antico-agulants in current use all target thrombin. These agents include recombi-nant hirudins, bivalirudin, and argatroban.

HEPARIN

Unfractionated heparin (UFH) is a highly sulfated negatively charged mucopolysaccharide that is heterogeneous with respect to molecular size, anticoagulant activity, and pharmacokinetic properties. UFH ranges in molecular weight from 3,000 to 30,000, with a mean of 15,000. UFH binds to AT through a unique pentasaccharide sequence producing a con-formational change that converts AT from a slow, progressive thrombin inhibitor to a rapid inhibitor of several coagulation enzymes. UFH then dissociates from the AT/enzyme complex and is reutilized. The parenteral anticoagulants low-molecular-weight heparin (LMWH) and fondaparinux exert their anticoagulant effects through similar mechanisms. After catalyz-ing the interaction between AT and the clotting enzyme, they also dissoci-ate from the AT/enzyme complex and can be reutilized. Unlike UFH, however, which inhibits thrombin and factor Xa equally well, LMWH has less antithrombin activity relative to its anti-factor Xa activity, and fonda-parinux only inhibits factor Xa.

Only about one-third of the UFH molecules possess the unique high affinity pentasaccharide sequence, and it is this fraction that is responsible for most of its anticoagulant effect.

The heparin/AT complex inactivates thrombin (factor IIa) and factors Xa, IXa, XIa, and XIIa. Thrombin and factor Xa are most sensitive to inhibition by heparin/AT, and thrombin is about tenfold more sensitive to inhibition than factor Xa. Heparin catalyzes AT-mediated thrombin inhibition by binding both to AT and to thrombin to form a ternary heparin/AT/thrombin complex. In contrast, to catalyze factor Xa inhibition by AT, heparin needs only to bind to AT via its high affinity pentasaccharide. Heparin chains consisting of fewer than 18 saccharide units are too short to bridge thrombin and AT. Consequently, these chains are unable to catalyze thrombin inhibition. However, as long as they possess a pentasaccharide, short heparin chains can catalyze inhibition of factor Xa by AT.

Heparin binds to a number of plasma-, platelet-, and endothelial-cell-derived proteins that compete with AT for heparin binding. Binding of heparin to plasma proteins contributes to the variability of the anticoagulant response among patients and to the heparin resistance seen in some patients with thromboembolic disorders.

Heparin also binds to macrophages where it is internalized, depolymerized, and metabolized into smaller and less sulfated forms. At low concentrations, it is cleared rapidly by a saturable cellular mechanism. At higher concentrations, it is cleared by a slower non-saturable renal clearance mechanism. At therapeutic concentrations, a major proportion of the heparin is cleared by the rapid saturable mechanism.

This complex mechanism of heparin clearance explains why the apparent biologic half-life of heparin increases from 30 to 60 to 150 minutes with intravenous (IV) boluses of 25, 100, and 400 U/kg of heparin, respectively. Heparin has decreased bioavailability when administered subcutaneously in low doses but has approximately 90% bioavailability when administered by subcutaneous (SC) injection in high therapeutic doses (eg, 35,000 U per 24 hours). LMWH exhibits less protein and cellular binding and, as a consequence, has a more predictable dose response, better bioavailability, and a longer plasma half-life. Fondaparinux has even less non-specific protein binding than LMWH, has excellent bioavailability and a predictable dose response.

As with all anticoagulants, the risk of heparin-associated bleeding increases with dosage. The risk of heparin-associated bleeding also increases during and after recent surgery, trauma, invasive procedures, and in patients with concomitant hemostatic defects.

There is a relationship between the dose of heparin administered and its efficacy. Therefore, to achieve efficacy, the dose of heparin is adjusted, usually by monitoring with the activated partial thromboplastin time (APTT), or when very high doses are given, by activated clotting time (ACT). These tests are sensitive mainly to antithrombin effects of heparin.

A less intense anticoagulant effect is required to prevent venous thrombosis with heparin than to treat established thrombosis. Low-dose heparin, 5,000 units subcutaneously twice or three times daily, is highly effective in preventing venous thrombosis in moderate-risk patients and is administered without laboratory monitoring.

A rapid therapeutic heparin effect is achieved in most patients by commencing with a loading dose. Initial dosing of heparin for VTE is weight-based—80 U/kg bolus and 18 U/kg/h infusion, which is roughly equivalent to a loading dose of 5,000 units and an infusion of 32,000 U per 24-hour infusion in a 70 kg person. Doses of heparin given to treat coronary thrombosis syndromes are lower than those typically used to treat VTE; the recommended dose is a bolus of 60 to 70 U/kg (maximum 5,000 U) and infusion of 12 to 15 U/kg/h (maximum 1,000 U/h) for unstable angina and non–ST-segment elevation myocardial infarction. Lower doses—60 U/kg bolus (maximum 4,000 U), 12 U/kg infusion (maximum 1,000 U/h)—are recommended in patients receiving recombinant tissue plasminogen activator (alteplase) for acute ST-segment elevation myocardial infarction.

In addition to hemorrhagic complications, UFH can be complicated by heparin-induced thrombocytopenia, by skin reactions after subcutaneous injections and, uncommonly, by osteoporosis and by hypersensitivity reactions. Heparin therapy can also cause elevations of serum transaminases. This phenomenon is benign and not associated with liver disease.

Heparin is effective for the prevention and treatment of VTE, for the early treatment of patients with unstable angina and acute myocardial infarction, for the treatment of patients who have cardiac surgery under cardiopulmonary bypass, and for patients having coronary angioplasty.

The anticoagulant effect of UFH can be rapidly reversed by intravenous protamine sulfate. One milligram of protamine sulfate will neutralize approximately 100 U of heparin.

LOW-MOLECULAR-WEIGHT HEPARIN

Low-molecular-weight heparins are derived from UFH by chemical or enzymatic depolymerization. LMWHs are about one-third the molecular weight of UFH, with a mean molecular weight of 4,000 to 6,000 and a range of 2,000 to 10,000 and, like UFH, LMWHs are heterogeneous in size. Reduction in molecular size is responsible for a change in the anticoagulant profile, an improvement in bioavailability and pharmacokinetics, and a reduction in the risk of osteopenia and heparin-induced thrombocytopenia.

Like UFH, LMWHs achieve their major anticoagulant effect by binding to AT through a unique pentasaccharide sequence. Less than

50% of different LMWH preparations have pentasaccharide-containing fragments with 18 or more saccharide units. Therefore, compared with UFH, which has a ratio of anti-factor Xa to anti-factor IIa activity of approximately 1:1, the various commercial LMWHs have anti-factor Xa to anti-factor IIa ratios varying between 4:1 and 2:1, depending on their molecular size distribution.

The plasma recoveries and pharmacokinetics of LMWHs differ from UFH because of differences in their respective binding properties to plasma proteins and cells. LMWHs bind much less avidly to heparin-binding proteins than UFH, a property that contributes to their superior bioavailability at low-doses and their more predictable anticoagulant response. LMWHs have a longer plasma half-life than UFH, and their clearance is dose-independent. LMWH is cleared in the urine, and its biologic half-life increases in patients with renal failure. Therefore, dosing can be problematic in severe renal insufficiency. In the setting of severe renal insufficiency when therapeutic anticoagulation is required, use of UFH avoids the problems associated with impaired clearance of LMWH preparations. If, however, LMWH is chosen, anti-factor Xa monitoring and/or dose reduction should be done to ensure there is no accumulation. LMWHs are typically administered in fixed doses for thromboprophylaxis, or in total-body-weight–adjusted doses when used to obtain a therapeutic effect. Laboratory monitoring is not generally necessary, but monitoring should be considered in patients with renal failure or severe obesity.

LMWHs are effective in the prevention and treatment of venous thrombosis and in the treatment of patients with unstable angina and non–Q-wave infarction. LMWHs have a number of advantages over heparin. Their use is associated with a lower incidence of heparin-induced thrombocytopenia and heparin-induced osteoporosis. Since they have a longer plasma half-life and a more predictable anticoagulant response than heparin, LMWHs can be administered once daily and without laboratory monitoring. This latter property is particularly useful for the out-of-hospital management of patients with venous thrombosis or unstable angina. There is no proven method for neutralizing LMWH, but protamine sulfate neutralizes a variable portion of the anti-factor Xa activity of LMWH.

FONDAPARINUX

Fondaparinux is a synthetic analog of the natural AT-binding pentasaccharide found in heparin and LMWH. Based on its modified structure, it has both a greater affinity for AT than the natural pentasaccharide and a longer half-life. Fondaparinux inactivates factor Xa in an AT-dependent manner, but, because it is too short to bridge AT to thrombin, fondaparinux does not increase the rate of thrombin inhibition by AT.

After subcutaneous injection, fondaparinux is rapidly and completely absorbed. It has a terminal half-life of 17 hours in young subjects and 21 hours in elderly volunteers, and is excreted unchanged in the urine. Fondaparinux exhibits linear pharmacokinetics and shows minimal non-specific binding to plasma proteins. Most of the compound is bound to AT, a property that accounts for its long half-life.

Fondaparinux is administered subcutaneously once daily in fixed doses without laboratory monitoring. The dose differs depending on the indication: for thromboprophylaxis, 2.5 mg once daily; for treatment of acute coronary syndromes, 2.5 mg once daily; and the drug is given at a dose of 7.5 mg for patients with a body weight of 50 to 100 kg for treatment of deep vein thrombosis (DVT, also called venous thrombosis or deep venous thrombosis) or pulmonary embolism. The dose is decreased to 5 mg for patients weighing less than 50 kg and increased to 10 mg in those weighing more than 100 kg. Fondaparinux is cleared in the urine and contraindicated in patients with renal insufficiency [creatinine clearance (CrCl) < 30 mL/min].

Fondaparinux has low affinity for platelet factor 4 PF4 and, therefore, does not cross-react with heparin-induced thrombocytopenia (HIT) antibodies. There have been no convincing reports of HIT with fondaparinux, and this agent has been used successfully to treat HIT patients. Results of in vitro studies using cultured osteoblasts suggest that fondaparinux will have minimal or no effects on bone metabolism.

Fondaparinux is effective for the following clinical situations: for prevention of venous thrombosis in high-risk orthopedic surgery, in general surgery and high-risk medical patients; for treatment of venous thrombosis and pulmonary embolism; and for treatment of patients with acute coronary insufficiency [both non–ST-elevation myocardial infarction (MI) and ST-elevation MI].

Fondaparinux does not bind to protamine sulfate, the antidote for heparin. If uncontrollable bleeding occurs with fondaparinux, recombinant factor VIIa may be effective.

DANAPAROID SODIUM

Danaparoid is a mixture of glycosaminoglycans (heparan sulfate, dermatan sulfate and chondroitin sulfate), and acts as an anticoagulant primarily by catalyzing the inhibition of factor Xa in an AT-dependent fashion. The drug has low specific anti-factor Xa activity. Based on anti-factor Xa levels, danaparoid has a half-life of approximately 25 hours.

Currently, the use of danaparoid is limited to the management of patients with HIT. Danaparoid does not prolong the international normalized ratio (INR). This property facilitates monitoring when transitioning HIT patients from danaparoid to vitamin K antagonists (VKAs). The long half-life of danaparoid is a disadvantage if patients require urgent surgery or invasive procedures. It also is problematic if patients have serious bleeding because there is no antidote for danaparoid.

DIRECT THROMBIN INHIBITORS

In contrast to indirect anticoagulants, which require a plasma cofactor to exert their activity, direct thrombin inhibitors have intrinsic activity because they bind to thrombin and block its enzymatic activity. The currently approved direct thrombin inhibitors are hirudin, bivalirudin, and argatroban.

Hirudin is a 65-amino-acid polypeptide now available in recombinant forms. Two recombinant forms of hirudin, known as lepirudin and desirudin, are currently approved for clinical use in North America and in Europe, respectively. Lepirudin is licensed for treatment of thrombosis-complicating HIT, whereas desirudin is approved in Europe for postoperative thromboprophylaxis in patients undergoing elective hip arthroplasty.

Hirudin is a bivalent thrombin inhibitor that binds both to the active site of thrombin and to exosite 1, the substrate-binding site, to form high affinity stoichiometric complexes with thrombin that are essentially irreversible.

The plasma half-life of hirudin is 60 minutes after intravenous injection and 120 minutes after subcutaneous injection. Hirudin is cleared via the kidneys, and the drug accumulates in patients with renal insufficiency. The dose of hirudin must be reduced when the creatinine clearance is less than 60 mL/min, and the drug is contraindicated in patients with renal failure.

The recommended dose of intravenous lepirudin for HIT is 0.15 mg/kg/h with or without an initial bolus of 0.4 mg/kg. The anticoagulant effect of lepirudin in this setting is monitored by using the APTT, and the dose is adjusted to achieve a target APTT ratio of 1.5:2.5.

When given for thromboprophylaxis after elective hip replacement surgery, desirudin is given subcutaneously at a dose of 15 mg twice daily. Routine APTT monitoring is unnecessary with this dose of desirudin.

Antibodies against hirudin develop in up to 40% of patients treated with lepirudin. Although most of these antibodies have no clinical impact, some can prolong the plasma half-life of lepirudin, resulting in drug accumulation. In addition, anaphylaxis can occur if patients with antibodies are re-exposed to hirudin. Consequently, an alternative anticoagulant should be used in HIT patients who have previously been treated with hirudin.

Bivalirudin is a 20-amino-acid synthetic polypeptide analog of hirudin. Like hirudin, it is a bivalent inhibitor that forms a 1:1 stoichiometric complex with thrombin. However, unlike hirudin, once bound, thrombin cleaves the proline-arginine (Pro-Arg) bond within the amino terminal of bivalirudin, thereby allowing recovery of thrombin activity. Bivalirudin has a plasma half-life of 25 minutes after intravenous injection, and only 20% is excreted via the kidneys. Bivalirudin is licensed as an alternative to heparin in patients undergoing percutaneous coronary interventions. The currently recommended dose is a bolus of 0.7 mg/kg followed by an infusion of 1.75 mg/kg/h for the duration of the procedure. Bivalirudin is also licensed as an alternative to heparin in HIT patients (with or without thrombosis) who require percutaneous coronary interventions. The drug is also being explored as an alternative to heparin in patients undergoing cardiopulmonary bypass surgery. In contrast to hirudin, bivalirudin is not immunogenic.

Argatroban is a univalent competitive inhibitor of thrombin that binds non-covalently to the active site of thrombin to form a reversible complex. The plasma half-life of argatroban is 45 minutes. It is metabolized in the liver via the cytochrome P450 3A4/5 enzyme system. Consequently, argatroban must be used with caution in patients with hepatic dysfunction. Argatroban is particularly useful in HIT patients with severe renal impairment.

Argatroban is licensed for treatment and prevention of HIT-associated thrombosis and for anticoagulation during percutaneous coronary interventions when heparin is contraindicated because of a recent history of HIT. Argatroban is given as a continuous intravenous infusion at a dose of 2 µg/kg/h, and the dose is adjusted to maintain the APTT ratio in the 1.5 to 2.5 range.

Although not ideal, the APTT is used to monitor therapy with direct thrombin inhibitors. The ecarin clotting time yields a more linear dose response than the APTT, but this test is not widely available and has not been standardized.

All of the direct thrombin inhibitors increase the INR and, therefore, can complicate monitoring when transitioning to vitamin K antagonists. The effect on the INR is most marked with argatroban. To overcome this problem, the INR can be measured after stopping the argatroban infusion for several hours or to monitor the vitamin K antagonist with a chromogenic factor X assay.

There are no specific antidotes for direct thrombin inhibitors. Factor VIIa might be effective but its utility in patients treated with direct thrombin inhibitors has not been established. Hemodialysis or hemoperfusion can remove bivalirudin or argatroban. Dialysis using special dialysis membranes can clear hirudin.

RECOMMENDATIONS

Monitoring Antithrombotic Effect

1. In patients treated with LMWH, we recommend against routine coagulation monitoring **(Grade 1C)**. In pregnant women treated with therapeutic doses of LMWH, we recommend monitoring of anti-factor Xa levels **(Grade 1C)**.

Dosing and Monitoring in Special Situations

1. In obese patients given LMWH prophylaxis or treatment, we suggest weight-based dosing **(Grade 2C)**. In patients with severe renal insufficiency (CrCl < 30 mL/min) who require therapeutic anticoagulation, we suggest the use of UFH instead of LMWH **(Grade 2C)**. If LMWH is used in patients with severe renal insufficiency (CrCl < 30 mL/min) who require therapeutic anticoagulation, we suggest using 50% of the recommended dose **(Grade 2C)**.

Direct Thrombin Inhibitors

1. In patients who receive either lepirudin or desirudin and have renal insufficiency (CrCl < 60 mL/min but > 30 mL/min), we recommend that the dose be reduced and the drug be monitored using the APTT **(Grade 1C)**. In patients with a CrCl < 30 mL/min, we recommend against the use of lepirudin or desirudin **(Grade 1C)**. In patients who require anticoagulation and have previously received lepirudin or desirudin, we recommend against repeated use of these drugs because of the risk of anaphylaxis **(Grade 1C)**.

Monitoring of Direct Thrombin Inhibitors

1. In patients receiving argatroban who are being transitioned to a vitamin K antagonist, we suggest that factor X levels, measured using a chromogenic assay, be used to adjust the dose of the vitamin K antagonist **(Grade 2C)**.

3 PHARMACOLOGY AND MANAGEMENT OF VITAMIN K ANTAGONISTS

Oral anticoagulants are vitamin K antagonists (VKAs). VKAs produce their anticoagulant effect by interfering with the cyclic interconversion of vitamin K and its 2,3 epoxide (vitamin K epoxide). Inhibition of this process results in the production of hemostatically defective vitamin K-dependent coagulant proteins (prothrombin, factor VII, factor IX, and factor X).

Warfarin, a coumarin compound, is the most widely used oral anticoagulant in North America. The drug is administered orally and is rapidly and almost completely absorbed from the gastrointestinal tract. Both the efficacy and safety of warfarin are closely related to the anticoagulant response achieved. Since the dose–response relationship of warfarin varies widely among individuals, the dose must be monitored closely to prevent overdosing or underdosing. Laboratory monitoring is performed by measuring the prothrombin time (PT). The PT is responsive to depression of three of the four vitamin K-dependent procoagulant clotting factors (prothrombin and factors VII and X), which are reduced at a rate proportionate to their respective half-lives. During the first few days of warfarin therapy, the PT reflects primarily the depression of factor VII, which has a half-life of only about 6 hours. Subsequently, the PT is prolonged also by depression of factors X and II.

Commercial PT reagents vary in their responsiveness to coumarin-induced reduction in clotting factors. This problem is overcome by reporting the PT as the international normalized ratio (INR).

The reliability of monitoring is improved by having dosage controlled in anticoagulation management services and by using computer-assisted algorithms. The reliability of monitoring is also improved by educating patients about warfarin treatment and by ensuring there is good communication between the patient and the appropriate health professional. The convenience of monitoring can be increased by using point-of-care testing with portable finger-prick monitors. Some of these devices are as accurate as traditional automated methods using citrated plasma. Patient self-management with point-of-care monitors has also been shown to be reliable in selected patients.

EFFECTIVE LEVELS OF ANTICOAGULATION

VKAs are effective in the primary and secondary prevention of VTE; in the prevention of systemic arterial embolism in patients with tissue and mechanical prosthetic heart valves, or in those with atrial fibrillation (AF); in the prevention of recurrent systemic embolism in patients with AF; in the prevention of acute myocardial infarction in patients with peripheral arterial disease; and in the prevention of stroke, recurrent infarction, and death in patients with acute myocardial infarction. VKAs are also indicated in patients with valvular heart disease to prevent systemic arterial embolism, although their effectiveness has never been demonstrated by a randomized clinical trial. A moderate intensity INR (2.0 to 3.0) is effective for most indications. The possible exceptions are acute myocardial infarction, in which a higher INR level might be superior, and in primary prevention of myocardial infarction in high-risk patients in which a lower INR is effective. In addition, a lower INR range (1.5 to 2.0) is effective in patients with venous thrombosis who have received 6 months of full-dose treatment (INR 2.0 to 3.0), although the lower intensity is less effective than the higher intensity. Fixed-dose warfarin has reduced efficacy or none at all, depending on the indication. The optimal INR level for patients with prosthetic heart valves remains uncertain, although there is evidence that these patients do not require the very high intensities that were used in the past.

FACTORS INFLUENCING ANTICOAGULANT EFFECT OF VITAMIN K ANTAGONISTS

The anticoagulant effect of VKA can be influenced by genetic and environmental factors.

Genetic Factors

A number of mutations in the gene coding for enzymes involved in either the metabolism or the anticoagulant (pharmacodynamic) response to warfarin can influence the anticoagulant response to drugs. These include: (1) mutations in the gene encoding for the cytochrome P450 2C9 hepatic microsomal enzyme, which result in increased S-warfarin elimination half-life; (2) mutations for the gene coding for vitamin K oxide reductase complex 1 (VKORC1), which result in enzymes with varying warfarin-binding affinities and which are likely to be the cause of hereditary warfarin resistance; (3) mutations in the gene encoding for the factor IX propeptide, which causes selective reduction in factor IX during treatment with coumarin drugs.

Environmental Factors

Environmental factors include diet, concomitant drug use, patient compliance, inaccuracies in laboratory testing and reporting, poor communication between patient and physician, and inappropriately large changes in dose of warfarin in response to modest fluctuations in INR.

Concomitant medication with over-the-counter drugs, prescription drugs, and herbal remedies can influence the INR by augmenting or inhibiting the anticoagulant effect of VKA. Patients receiving warfarin therapy are also sensitive to fluctuating levels of dietary vitamin K, which is obtained predominantly from leafy green vegetables. Increased intake of dietary vitamin K occurs in patients on weight reduction diets (rich in green vegetables) and those treated with intravenous (IV) nutritional fluid supplements rich in vitamin K. The effects of warfarin can be potentiated in sick patients with poor vitamin K intake (particularly if they are treated with antibiotics and IV fluids without vitamin K supplementation) and in states of fat malabsorption. Hepatic dysfunction also potentiates the response to warfarin through impaired synthesis of coagulation factors. Hypermetabolic states produced by fever or hyperthyroidism increase the responsiveness to warfarin, probably by increasing the catabolism of vitamin K-dependent coagulation factors.

A number of drugs can increase the risk of warfarin-associated bleeding by inhibiting platelet function. Of these, aspirin [acetylsalicylic acid (ASA)] is the most important because it is present in many over-the-counter preparations and because it has a prolonged effect on hemostasis. Aspirin can also produce gastric erosions, which increase the risk of serious upper gastrointestinal bleeding.

Many other drugs have the potential to influence the effect of warfarin on hemostasis. Therefore, when treatment with any new drug is necessary in patients who are being treated with oral anticoagulants, the PT should be monitored every second day or so during the initial stages of combined drug therapy, with dose adjustments made as necessary.

PRACTICAL DOSING

If a rapid anticoagulant effect is required, heparin [or low-molecular-weight heparin (LMWH) or fondaparinux] and warfarin should be started at the same time and overlapped for at least 4 days. When the INR has been in the therapeutic range on two measurements approximately 24 hours apart, heparin is usually discontinued. The selection of the appropriate starting dose of warfarin is influenced by the clinical status of the patient. A starting dose of 5 mg is appropriate in hospitalized patients, but it is reasonable to use a starting dose of 7.5 to 10 mg in otherwise healthy people. A lower starting dose (5 mg or less) would be appropriate in patients at high risk of bleeding, in sick patients (particularly in those with liver disease or congestive heart failure), in the elderly, in patients with impaired nutrition and if treatment is not urgent. If treatment initiation is not urgent (eg, in chronic stable atrial fibrillation), warfarin administration, without concurrent heparin administration, can be commenced out-of-hospital with an anticipated maintenance dose of 4 to 5 mg/d.

MONITORING

In hospitalized patients, INR monitoring is usually performed daily until the therapeutic range has been achieved and maintained for at least 2 consecutive days, then two or three times weekly for 1 to 2 weeks, then less often, depending on the stability of INR results. In outpatients started on warfarin, initial monitoring may be reduced to every few days until a stable dose response has been achieved. When the INR response is stable, the frequency of testing can be reduced gradually to intervals as long as every 4 weeks, although there is evidence that testing more frequently than every 4 weeks will lead to a greater time in therapeutic range. If dose adjustments are required, the cycle of more frequent monitoring is repeated until a stable dose response is again achieved.

MANAGEMENT OF NONTHERAPEUTIC INR

Various options can be followed for the management of patients whose INR is outside the therapeutic range. Patients whose INR is just outside the therapeutic range can be managed by either adjusting the dose up or down in 5 to 20% increments based on the cumulative weekly dose of warfarin, or by more frequent monitoring—the latter with the expectation that the INR will return to therapeutic levels without a dosage change. High INR values, between 4.0 and 9.0, can be managed by stopping warfarin for a day or more, reducing the weekly dose and monitoring more frequently. However, in patients with a high risk for bleeding, or who are bleeding, a more active approach should be used to lower the INR more rapidly. The interventions include administering vitamin K_1; and infusing fresh frozen plasma, prothrombin concentrates, or recombinant factor VIIa. If a decision is made to use vitamin K_1, it should be administered in a dose that will quickly lower the INR into a safe range without causing warfarin resistance when the VKA is restarted, and by a route that minimizes the risk of anaphylaxis. High doses of vitamin K_1, though effective, may lower the INR more than is necessary and lead to warfarin resistance for up to a week or more. Intravenous injection may be associated with anaphylactic reactions. The response to subcutaneous vitamin K_1 is less predictable than oral vitamin K_1, whereas oral administration is predictably effective, and has the advantages of safety and convenience. A dose range of 1.0 to 2.5 mg is effective when the INR is between 5.0 and 9.0, but larger doses (5 mg), are required to correct INR values over 9.0. Vitamin K_1 can also be administered by slow intravenous infusion when there is a greater urgency to reverse anticoagulation.

If continuing warfarin therapy is indicated after high doses of vitamin K_1, then heparin can be given until the effects of vitamin K_1 have been reversed and the patient becomes responsive to warfarin therapy.

MANAGEMENT OF VARIABLE INR LEVELS

The common causes of variable INR levels are poor patient compliance, inappropriate dosing adjustments to mild fluctuations in the INR, and drugs or foods that influence the anticoagulant response to warfarin. There is also evidence that, in patients with poor or variable vitamin K intake, more stable anticoagulation can be achieved by using supplemental vitamin K. Therefore, fixed low doses of vitamin K supplements can be considered in carefully screened patients with a variable INR response

RECOMMENDATIONS

Initiation and Maintenance Dosing
1. In patients beginning VKA therapy, we recommend the initiation of oral anticoagulation with doses between 5 and 10 mg for the first 1 or 2 days for most individuals, with subsequent dosing based on the INR response **(Grade 1B)**. At the present time, for patients beginning VKA therapy, without evidence from randomized trials, we suggest against the use of pharmacogenetics-based initial dosing to individualize warfarin dosing **(Grade 2C)**.

Initiation of Anticoagulation in the Elderly or Other Populations
1. In the elderly, or in patients who are debilitated, malnourished, have congestive heart failure, have liver disease, have had recent major surgery, or are taking medications known to increase the sensitivity to warfarin (eg, amiodarone), we recommend the use of a starting dose of ≤ 5 mg **(Grade 1C)**, with subsequent dosing based on the INR response.

Frequency of Monitoring
1. In patients beginning VKA therapy, we suggest that INR monitoring should be started after the initial two or three doses of oral anticoagulation therapy **(Grade 2C)**.

2. For patients who are receiving a stable dose of oral anticoagulants, we suggest monitoring at an interval of no longer than every 4 weeks **(Grade 2C)**.

Management of Nontherapeutic INRs

1. For patients with INRs above the therapeutic range, but < 5.0 and with no significant bleeding, we recommend lowering the dose or omitting a dose, monitoring more frequently, and resuming therapy at an appropriately adjusted dose when the INR is at a therapeutic level. If only minimally above therapeutic range, or associated with a transient causative factor, no dose reduction may be required **(all Grade 1C)**.

2. For patients with INRs of ≥ 5.0 but < 9.0 and no significant bleeding, we recommend omitting the next one or two doses, monitoring more frequently, and resuming therapy at an appropriately adjusted dose when the INR is at a therapeutic level **(Grade 1C)**. Alternatively, we suggest omitting a dose and administering vitamin K orally (1 to 2.5 mg), particularly if the patient is at increased risk of bleeding **(Grade 2A)**. If more rapid reversal is required because the patient requires urgent surgery, we suggest vitamin K orally (≤ 5 mg) with the expectation that a reduction of the INR will occur in 24 hours. If the INR is still high, we suggest additional vitamin K orally (1 to 2 mg) **(Grade 2C)**.

3. For patients with INRs of > 9.0 and no significant bleeding, we recommend holding warfarin therapy and administering a higher dose of vitamin K orally (2.5 to 5 mg), with the expectation that the INR will be reduced substantially in 24 to 48 hours **(Grade 1B)**. Clinicians should monitor the INR more frequently, administer additional vitamin K if necessary, and resume therapy at an appropriately adjusted dose when the INR reaches the therapeutic range.

4. In patients with serious bleeding and elevated INR, regardless of the magnitude of the elevation, we recommend holding warfarin therapy and giving vitamin K (10 mg) by slow IV infusion supplemented with fresh frozen plasma, prothrombin complex concentrate, or recombinant factor VIIa, depending on the urgency of the situation. We recommend repeating vitamin K administration every 12 hours for persistent INR elevation **(all Grade 1C)**.

5. In patients with life-threatening bleeding (eg, intracranial hemorrhage) and elevated INR, regardless of the magnitude of the elevation, we recommend holding warfarin therapy and administering fresh frozen plasma, prothrombin complex concentrate or recombinant factor VIIa supplemented with vitamin K (10 mg) by slow IV infusion, repeated, if necessary, depending on the INR **(Grade 1C)**.

6. In patients with mild to moderately elevated INRs without major bleeding, we recommend that, when vitamin K is to be given, it be administered orally rather than subcutaneously **(Grade 1A)**.

Management of Variable INRs

1. For patients on chronic warfarin therapy with a variable INR response not attributable to any of the usual known causes for instability, we suggest a trial of daily low-dose oral vitamin K (100 to 200 µg) with close monitoring of the INR and warfarin dose adjustment to counter an initial lowering of the INR in response to vitamin K **(Grade 2B)**.

Management of INRs in the Antiphospholipid Syndrome

1. In patients who have a lupus inhibitor, who have no additional risk factors, and no lack of response to therapy, we recommend a therapeutic target INR of 2.5 (INR range: 2.0 to 3.0) **(Grade 1A)**. In patients who have recurrent thromboembolic events with a therapeutic INR, we suggest a target INR of 3.0 (INR range: 2.5 to 3.5) **(Grade 2C)**.

Optimal Management of Vitamin K Antagonist Therapy

1. For health care providers who manage oral anticoagulation therapy, we recommend they do so in a systematic and coordinated fashion, incorporating patient education, systematic INR testing, tracking, follow-up, and good patient communication of results and dosing decisions as occurs in an anticoagulation management service **(Grade 1B)**.

Patient Self-Testing and Patient Self-Management

1. Patient self-monitoring (PSM) is a choice made by patients and health care providers that depends on many factors. In patients who are suitably selected and trained, patient self-testing or PSM is an effective alternative treatment model. We suggest that such therapeutic management be implemented where suitable **(Grade 2B)**.

4 ANTIPLATELET DRUGS

The platelet-active drugs that are effective in prevention and treatment of arterial thrombosis are aspirin, ticlopidine, clopidogrel, dipyridamole, abciximab, and the small-molecular-weight glycoprotein (GP) IIb-IIIa inhibitors tirofiban and eptifibatide. Since the last report, new information has been published suggesting that (1) bleeding risks with aspirin increase with aspirin dose; (2) coxibs and some nonsteroidal anti-inflammatory drugs (NSAIDs) increase cardiovascular risk; (3) the combination of aspirin and clopidogrel is no more effective than either drug alone in stroke; and (4) the combination of aspirin and clopidogrel is less effective than warfarin in patients with atrial fibrillation.

ASPIRIN

Aspirin [acetylsalicylic acid (ASA)] is an effective antithrombotic agent that inhibits the production of thromboxane A_2 (TXA_2), a potent inducer of platelet aggregation and vasoconstriction, by inhibiting platelet cyclooxygenase (COX-1). Aspirin prevents vascular death by approximately 15% and nonfatal vascular events by about 30%.

Mechanism of Action of Aspirin

Aspirin permanently inactivates prostaglandin H-synthase (PGHS)-1 and -2 (also referred to as COX-1 and COX-2). The COX isozymes catalyze the conversion of arachidonic acid to prostaglandin H_2 (PGH_2), which is the precursor of a variety of prostaglandins, including thromboxane [TXA_2 and prostacyclin (PGI_2)]. Aspirin is approximately 50- to 100-fold more potent in inhibiting platelet COX-1 than COX-2 in monocytes and other inflammatory cells. Consequently, the COX-2–dependent anti-inflammatory effects of aspirin require larger doses of the drug because of (1) a decreased sensitivity of COX-2 to aspirin, and (2) a much more short-lived inhibitory effect of aspirin on inflammatory cells because these nucleated cells rapidly resynthesize the enzyme. Aspirin produces a permanent defect in TXA_2-dependent function in platelets since these non-nucleated cells are incapable of synthesizing new COX-1. Aspirin also inactivates COX-1 in relatively mature megakaryocytes. Since only 10% of the platelet pool is replenished each day, once-a-day dosing of aspirin is able to maintain virtually complete inhibition of platelet TXA_2 production.

Human platelets and vascular endothelial cells process PGH_2 to produce TXA_2 and PGI_2, respectively. TXA_2 induces platelet aggregation and vasoconstriction, whereas PGI_2 inhibits platelet aggregation and induces vasodilatation. TXA_2 is mostly a COX-1–derived platelet product, whereas vascular PGI_2 can derive from both COX-1 and COX-2. Low, and even moderate, doses of aspirin do not inhibit PGI_2 synthesis substantially because the effect of aspirin on endothelial cell-derived COX-1 is short-lived, and COX-2 is largely insensitive to aspirin inhibition at conventional antiplatelet doses. There is increasing evidence that suppression of PGI_2 formation increases the risk of thrombosis. Thus, studies with mice deficient in the gene encoding the PGI_2 receptor, and the observation of the cardiovascular toxicity associated with COX-2 inhibitors, support the importance of this prostanoid in the prevention of arterial thrombosis.

There is evidence that COX-2 inhibitors produce a two- to three fold increased risk of vascular events. There is also evidence that traditional NSAIDs are associated with an increased risk of vascular events, likely through inhibition of PGI_2 formation, although naproxen appears to be free of this untoward effect.

Effects of Aspirin Not Related to TXA$_2$

Aspirin has been reported to have effects on hemostasis that are unrelated to its ability to inactivate platelet COX-1. These include dose-dependent, non-specific inhibition of platelet function, enhancement of fibrinolysis, and suppression of plasma coagulation. None of these effects have been shown to contribute to the antithrombotic effect of aspirin. In contrast, there is overwhelming evidence that the antithrombotic effect of aspirin is largely derived from its ability to inhibit COX-1 in platelets.

Pharmacokinetics of Aspirin

Aspirin is rapidly absorbed in the stomach and upper intestine and has a short half-life (15 to 20 minutes) in the human circulation. Peak plasma levels occur 30 to 40 minutes after aspirin ingestion, and inhibition of platelet function is evident by 1 h. In contrast, it can take up to 3 to 4 h to reach peak plasma levels after administration of enteric-coated aspirin. If only enteric-coated tablets are available, and a rapid effect is required, the tablets should be chewed. The oral bioavailability of regular aspirin tablets is approximately 40 to 50% over a wide range of doses. A considerably lower bioavailability has been reported for enteric-coated tablets and sustained-release, microencapsulated preparations. Because platelet COX-1 is acetylated in the pre-systemic circulation, the antiplatelet effect of aspirin is largely independent of systemic bioavailability.

Aspirin reduces the incidence of myocardial infarction and/or death in the following groups of patients: those with silent myocardial ischemia or with stable angina; those with unstable angina and non–Q-wave infarction; those with acute myocardial infarction; in patients after angioplasty and aortocoronary bypass surgery; and in patients with cerebrovascular disease.

There is also evidence that aspirin prevents myocardial infarction in asymptomatic males and females over the age of 50 years, although the relative risks and benefits in asymptomatic individuals are less certain than in those with overt evidence of atherosclerotic vascular disease. Therefore, the risks of aspirin must be weighed carefully against the small benefits in asymptomatic persons. For patients with acute myocardial infarction, prior infarction, or prior stroke, aspirin prevents between 35 and 40 events per 1,000 patients treated. In contrast, when used in asymptomatic patients, aspirin prevents only four events per 1,000 patients treated. Low-dose aspirin does not reduce maternal and fetal complications in pregnant women with hypertension, past or present preeclampsia, renal disease, or history of intrauterine growth retardation. The addition of aspirin (100 mg) to warfarin increases the efficacy of warfarin in preventing systemic embolism and vascular death in patients with mechanical prosthetic heart valves but at an increased risk of bleeding. Other effective aspirin combinations are (1) aspirin and dipyridamole in patients with stroke; (2) low-dose aspirin with heparin to prevent recurrent miscarriages in pregnant women with antiphospholipid antibody syndrome; (3) aspirin and clopidogrel to prevent acute thrombosis of coronary stents and in patients with unstable angina or non–ST-elevation myocardial infarction.

Aspirin produces a very small increase in the risk of cerebral hemorrhage, which is more than overcome by its much greater beneficial effects in reducing ischemic stroke in high-risk patients.

The antithrombotic effects of a range of doses of aspirin have been evaluated. Aspirin is effective when used in doses between 50 and 1,500 mg/d, and there is no evidence that low doses (50 to 100 mg/d) are less effective than high doses (650 to 1,500 mg/d). Doses of approximately 300 mg/d produce fewer gastrointestinal (GI) side effects than doses of approximately 1,200 mg/d. In the Clopidogrel in Unstable Angina to Prevent Recurrent Events (CURE) trial, patients with acute coronary syndromes receiving aspirin at ≤ 100 mg daily had the lowest rate of major or life-threatening bleeding complications without any loss in efficacy. Since the GI toxicity of aspirin and bleeding appear to be dose-related, the lowest dose of aspirin shown effective in each clinical setting is recommended in all clinical conditions in which antiplatelet prophylaxis has a favorable benefit/risk profile.

There has been recent interest in the phenomenon of aspirin-resistant TXA_2 biosynthesis. Potential mechanisms that might be responsible for aspirin-resistant TXA_2 biosynthesis include (1) the transient expression of COX-2 in newly formed platelets in clinical settings of enhanced platelet turn-over; (2) extra-platelet sources of TXA_2 (eg, monocyte/macrophage COX-2); (3) concomitant administration of a traditional NSAID (eg, ibuprofen) which may interfere with the irreversible inactivation of platelet COX-1 by aspirin. The clinical relevance of aspirin "resistance," particularly as a mechanism of aspirin failure, remains to be established.

DIPYRIDAMOLE

Dipyridamole is a pyrimido-pyrimidine derivative with vasodilator and antiplatelet properties. Dipyridamole inhibits platelet function by elevating platelet cyclic adenosine monophosphate (AMP) levels by (1) inhibition of cyclic nucleotide phosphodiesterase, the enzyme that degrades cyclic AMP to 5^1-AMP; and (2) blockade of the uptake of adenosine, thereby stimulating platelet adenylyl cyclase.

The absorption of dipyridamole from conventional formulations is quite variable and may result in low systemic bioavailability of the drug. A modified-release formulation of dipyridamole with improved bioavailability has been developed and has been evaluated in association with low-dose aspirin. Dipyridamole is eliminated primarily by biliary excretion as a glucuronide conjugate and is subject to enterohepatic recirculation. A terminal half-life of 10 hours has been reported. This is consistent with the twice-daily regimen used in recent clinical studies.

Although the efficacy of dipyridamole, alone or in combination with aspirin, has been questioned in the past, the results of the Second European Stroke Prevention Study (ESPS-2) and the European/Australasian Stroke Prevention in Reversible Ischaemia Trial (ESPRIT), both trials in patients with ischemic cerebrovascular disease, indicate that the combination of modified-release dipyridamole and low-dose aspirin is more effective for this indication than aspirin alone.

The combination of modified-release dipyridamole and low-dose aspirin has been recently approved by the US Food and Drug Administration (FDA).

THIENOPYRIDINES

Ticlopidine and clopidogrel are structurally related thienopyridines that selectively inhibit adenosine diphosphate (ADP)-induced platelet aggregation. Both drugs derive their antiplatelet effect through their hepatic transformation in vivo to (an) active metabolite(s). Platelets contain three receptors for ADP: a ligand-gated ion channel ($P2X_1$), a G-protein–linked receptor ($P2Y_1$), and a third, less–well-characterized receptor ($P2Y_{12}$). Clopidogrel and ticlopidine induce irreversible (permanent) alterations to this third ADP receptor that is postulated to mediate the inhibition of stimulated adenylyl cyclase activity. The irreversible modification of this ADP receptor site has been attributed to the formation of (a) disulfide bridge(s) between the reactive thiol group of the active metabolite of clopidogrel and that of (a) cysteine residue(s) of the platelet $P2Y_{12}$ receptor. The onset of action of the thienopyridines is delayed until the compounds are biotransformed to their active metabolites, and the recovery of platelet function is delayed until the metabolites are cleared and new unaffected platelets enter the circulation.

Up to 90% of a single oral dose of ticlopidine is rapidly absorbed in humans. Peak plasma concentrations occur 1 to 3 h after a single oral dose of 250 mg. Ticlopidine is transformed rapidly and extensively to a variety of metabolites, one of which (the 2-keto derivative) is more potent than the parent compound in inhibiting ADP-induced platelet aggregation.

Ticlopidine is an effective antithrombotic agent, but its clinical benefit is offset by two important side effects: hypercholesterolemia and neutropenia. Ticlopidine has also been associated with thrombocytopenia, aplastic anemia, and thrombotic thrombocytopenic purpura (TTP). Ticlopidine is approved for clinical use in patients with cerebral ischemia when aspirin has failed, cannot be tolerated, or is contraindicated, although this limitation does not apply to all countries where the drug is registered.

Several studies have demonstrated the superiority of the combination of ticlopidine and aspirin compared with aspirin alone, or aspirin plus warfarin, in preventing thrombotic complications after coronary artery stent placement. However, the better safety profile of clopidogrel has resulted in the substitution of clopidogrel for ticlopidine in many centers for this indication

Clopidogrel is rapidly absorbed and metabolized to its carboxylic acid derivative, SR 26334. The plasma elimination half-life of SR 26334 is approximately 8 hours. The onset of the inhibition of platelet aggregation with clopidogrel is more rapid than that observed with ticlopidine. Thus, inhibition of platelet aggregation is detectable as soon as 2 hours after an oral loading dosing of 300 mg and remains relatively stable up to 48 hours. Inhibition of ADP-induced platelet aggregation occurs in a dose-dependent fashion with an apparent ceiling effect of 40% inhibition after a single oral loading dose. Upon repeated daily administration of low doses, there is cumulative inhibition of platelet function with a return to normal 7 days after the last dose of clopidogrel.

The optimal timing and size of the loading dose for achieving a prompt antiplatelet effect in the acute setting is still under investigation, and doses up to 600 mg are currently being used as a loading dose of clopidogrel prior to percutaneous coronary intervention (PCI). In one recent trial in moderate-risk patients, the clinical outcome was similar, with or without abciximab, when a 600 mg loading dose of clopidogrel prior to PCI.

Patients exhibit considerable inter-individual variability to the ADP-inhibiting effects of clopidogrel on platelets. Three separate studies suggest that concurrent treatment with lipophilic statins that are substrates of Cytochrome P3A4 (CYP3A4) (eg, atorvastatin and simvastatin) can interfere with the inhibitory effects of clopidogrel on platelet function. Many drugs are metabolized by CYP3A4, so it is possible that other drugs may modify the systemic bioavailability of the active metabolite of clopidogrel and affect its clinical efficacy.

In the Clopidogrel versus Aspirin in Patients at Risk of Ischaemic Events study (CAPRIE), clopidogrel was shown to be more effective than aspirin in patients with atherothrombosis. Dual antiplatelet therapy with the combination of aspirin and clopidogrel has also been shown to be more effective than aspirin alone in a number of clinical trials in acute coronary syndrome (ACS) patients. In contrast, dual antiplatelet therapy with aspirin and clopidogrel was not more effective than clopidogrel alone in patients who suffered a recent ischemic stroke or transient ischemic attack (TIA). Furthermore, dual antiplatelet therapy with clopidogrel and aspirin was not more effective than aspirin alone in patients at high risk for atherothrombotic events, and it was less effective than warfarin in patients with atrial fibrillation.

INTEGRIN $\alpha_{IIB}\beta_3$ (GPIIB-IIIA) RECEPTOR ANTAGONISTS

The expression of functionally active integrin $\alpha_{IIb}\beta_3$ (GPIIb-IIIa) on the platelet surface is the final common pathway of platelet aggregation. The GPIIb-IIIa antagonists include monoclonal antibodies against the receptor, synthetic RGD- or Lys-Gly-Asp sequence (KGD) containing peptides, and peptidomimetic and nonpeptide RGD mimetics that compete with fibrinogen and von Willebrand factor for occupancy of the integrin platelet receptor.

Abciximab
Abciximab (ReoPro), the first GPIIb-IIIa antagonist developed for clinical use, is a mouse/human chimeric 7E3 Fab antibody. Platelet aggregation is nearly completely abolished when approximately 80% of the receptors are blocked. Abciximab is unique among the GPIIb-IIIa antagonists in also blocking the $\alpha_v\beta_3$ receptor and binding to an activated form of the leukocyte $\alpha M\beta2$ receptor; it is unclear whether any of abciximab's antithrombotic effects are due to inhibition of these receptors.

Following IV bolus administration, free plasma concentrations decrease rapidly (initial half-life of about 30 minutes) as a result of rapid binding to platelet GPIIb-IIIa receptors. Platelet aggregation in response to 20 M Molar ADP returns to 50% of baseline within 24 hours in most patients and within 48 hours in nearly all patients. Small amounts of abciximab can be detected on circulating platelets as late as 14 days after administration, presumably as a result of antibody redistribution from platelet to platelet.

Tirofiban
Tirofiban (MK-383; Aggrastat) is a nonpeptide derivative of tyrosine that selectively inhibits the GPIIb-IIIa receptor. When administered to humans

at 0.15 g/kg/min for 4 hours, tirofiban produced a 2.5-fold increase in bleeding time and 97% inhibition of ADP-induced platelet aggregation. Its half-life in plasma is 1.6 hours. After stopping tirofiban therapy, within 4 hours, bleeding times return to normal, and inhibition of platelet aggregation declines to approximately 20%. When administered with aspirin, the bleeding time increased about 1.5-fold.

Eptifibatide

Eptifibatide (Integrilin) is a synthetic disulfide-linked cyclic heptapeptide. It is patterned after the KGD sequence found in the snake venom disintegrin obtained from *Sistrurus miliarius barbouri* (barbourin) and has high specificity for inhibition of binding to GPIIb-IIIa receptors. The elimination of eptifibatide depends principally on plasma clearance. Two hours after discontinuing an eptifibatide infusion, there is a substantial return of platelet function and return of more than half of the baseline aggregation response in all groups after 4 hours.

Efficacy and Safety

The efficacy and safety of abciximab and the small molecular weight antagonists have been demonstrated in patients undergoing percutaneous coronary intervention (PCI). Over 20,000 patients have been enrolled in nine studies of abciximab, eptifibatide, and tirofiban. The first of these phase 3 trials, the Evaluation of c7E3 to Prevent Ischemic Complications (EPIC) trial, resulted in approval in many countries for abciximab for PCI patients at high risk of developing ischemic complication. The c7E3 Antiplatelet Therapy in Unstable Refractory Angina (CAPTURE) trial demonstrated the efficacy of abciximab treatment 18 to 24 hours prior to PCI in patients with unstable angina refractory to conventional antithrombotic and antianginal therapy. The Evaluation in PTCA to Improve Long-Term Outcome with Abciximab GP IIb/IIIa Blockade (EPILOG) trial demonstrated the efficacy of abciximab in a broad patient population undergoing PCI, and the Evaluation of Platelet IIb/IIIa Inhibitor for Stenting Trial (EPISTENT) demonstrated that abciximab decreases the frequency of ischemic complications of PCI associated with stent insertion during the first 30 days.

A meta-analysis of all major randomized clinical trials of GPIIb-IIIa antagonists in patients with acute coronary syndromes who were not routinely scheduled to undergo early coronary revascularization reported a 9% reduction in the odds of death or myocardial infarction at 30 days. The 1% absolute difference in death or myocardial infarction was balanced by an absolute excess of 1% in major bleeding complications associated with GPIIb-IIIa antagonists versus control.

Abciximab was compared to tirofiban as treatment for PCI in the Do Tirofiban and Reopro Give Similar Efficacy Outcomes (TARGET) study. Abciximab treatment was found to be associated with a statistically significant lower rate of ischemic complications after 30 days; at 6 months, the differences were less apparent.

Oral GPIIb-IIIa Antagonists

Orally active nonpeptide GPIIb-IIIa inhibitors have been developed for long-term use. The results of these studies, which included over 40,000 patients who had recovered from acute coronary ischemia, have been disappointing. The consistent finding of these large-scale trials is that oral GPIIb-IIIa antagonists (xemilofiban, orbofiban, sibrafiban, and lotrafiban) are not more effective than aspirin or, when combined with aspirin, are not superior to placebo and may, in fact, increase mortality. Several mechanisms have been put forward to explain these results. One is that the poor oral bioavailability of these compounds, combined with a target of 50% inhibition of platelet aggregation, resulted in trivial antiplatelet activity in many patients. An alternative (or additional) explanation is that GPIIb-IIIa antagonists can activate platelets.

5 NEW ANTITHROMBOTIC DRUGS

Novel antithrombotic agents have been developed in an attempt to overcome the shortcomings of existing agents. Although aspirin and the thienopyridine clopidogrel are effective antithrombotic agents, resistance to usual doses of aspirin, as manifested by incomplete inhibition of platelet aggregation and/or thromboxane A_2 production, occurs in some patients. Likewise, resistance to clopidogrel, as manifested by weak or absent inhibition of platelet aggregation, occurs in some patients. In addition, clopidogrel has a delayed onset and offset of action that could be problematic in certain clinical situations. These limitations, plus the incomplete protection against thromboembolic events, have stimulated the development of novel antiplatelet agents.

New adenosine diphosphate (ADP) ($P2Y_{12}$) receptor antagonists and drugs that target protease activated receptor (PAR)-1, the major thrombin receptor on platelets, are under clinical development. The new ADP receptor antagonists have a more rapid onset and offset of action than clopidogrel and they are more potent.

The currently available anticoagulants are the parenteral agents, unfractionated heparin (UFH), low-molecular-weight heparin (LMWH), fondaparinux and direct thrombin inhibitors, and the oral coumarins. New parenteral anticoagulants include analog of fondaparinux with a longer half-life, plus direct inhibitors that target thrombin or factors Xa, VIIa, IXa and compounds that promote protein C activation. New oral anticoagulants include direct inhibitors of thrombin or factor Xa.

NEW ANTIPLATELET AGENTS

New antiplatelet agents in advanced stages of development target the thromboxane A_2, ADP, and thrombin receptors on platelets.

Thromboxane A_2 Receptor Antagonists

A selective orally active inhibitor of the thromboxane A_2 receptor on platelets, S18886 is being investigated for secondary prevention of stroke in a large phase II trial.

ADP Receptor Antagonists

New ADP receptor antagonists include prasugrel, a thienopyridine, and cangrelor and AZD6140, direct competitive inhibitors of $P2Y_{12}$.

Prasugrel

Prasugrel, a thienopyridine, is a prodrug like clopidogrel that requires hepatic conversion to express its antiplatelet activity by irreversibly inhibiting the $P2Y_{12}$ receptor. Prasugrel is rapidly absorbed from the gastrointestinal tract and is then hydrolyzed by esterases to an inactive metabolite that is then further metabolized by the hepatic cytochrome P450 (CYP) enzyme system to an active form. Absorption occurs with little intersubject variability and, based on its method of metabolism, it is proposed that prasugrel is less likely than clopidogrel to exhibit pharmacodynamic resistance. Although the onset of platelet inhibition is more rapid with prasugrel than it is with clopidogrel, both drugs have a delayed offset of action because they irreversibly inhibit their target receptor. A large phase III trial comparing prasugrel with clopidogrel in patients with ST-segment or non–ST-segment elevation MI has recently been completed. The results showed that prasugrel was more effective than clopidogrel, but at the cost of increased bleeding.

Cangrelor

Cangrelor, an ATP analog, is a competitive inhibitor of $P2Y_{12}$. It produces almost immediate inhibition of ADP-induced platelet aggregation after intravenous administration. The drug has a half-life of about 3 to 5 minutes. Cangrelor has been evaluated in a two-part phase II trial in patients undergoing PCI and is currently undergoing phase III evaluation in PCI patients.

AZD6140

AZD6140 is an orally active variant of cangrelor that acts as a direct competitive inhibitor of $P2Y_{12}$. Like cangrelor, AZD6140 does not require hepatic conversion to an active metabolite. AZD6140 produces rapid reversible inhibition of ADP-induced platelet aggregation, but it has to be administered twice daily.

When compared with clopidogrel in a small phase II study, AZD6140 produced more rapid and more potent inhibition of ADP-induced platelet aggregation. In a larger phase II study, AZ6140 produced similar rates of bleeding to clopidogrel. AZD6140 is currently being evaluated in phase III trials.

PAR-1 Antagonists

Human platelets contain PAR-1 and PAR-4, both of which can be activated by thrombin to cause platelet secretion and aggregation. PAR-1 is considered to be the major thrombin receptor on human platelets because affinity of PAR-1 for thrombin is 40-fold higher than that of PAR-4. Consequently, PAR-1 is activated by lower concentrations of thrombin than PAR-4.

Two orally active PAR-1 antagonists, SCH-530348 and E5555, are undergoing phase II clinical evaluation.

SCH-530348

SCH-530348 is a synthetic analog of an alkaloid isolated from the bark of Australian magnolia trees. The drug has excellent oral bioavailability, has a long half-life, and inhibits thrombin receptor activating peptides TRAP-induced platelet aggregation for up to 4 weeks. Promising results were reported with SCH-530348 in a randomized phase II in 573 patients who underwent percutaneous coronary intervention (PCI). All received aspirin, clopidogrel, and an anticoagulant (either heparin or bivalirudin). There was no increase in bleeding, and the primary efficacy endpoint (death and major adverse cardiovascular events) occurred in 8.6% and 5.9%, respectively. SCH-530348 is now undergoing phase III evaluation in a wide range of ACS patients.

E5555

E5555 is a reversible PAR-1 antagonist that exhibits good oral bioavailability and is rapidly absorbed. The antiplatelet effects of E5555 persist for about 1 week Like SCH-530348, E5555 does not appear to prolong the bleeding time when administered to healthy volunteers. Phase II trials evaluating E5555 in patients with ACS are under way.

NEW ANTICOAGULANTS

Inhibitors of Factor VIIa/Tissue Factor Complex
All drugs in this category that have reached phase II or III clinical testing are parenteral agents.

Tifacogin
Tifacogin is a recombinant form of tissue factory pathway inhibitor that has been evaluated in patients with sepsis. The drug has a half-life of minutes and is cleared by the liver. After a successful phase II trial with sepsis patients, the drug was evaluated in a phase III trial in 1,754 severe sepsis patients. The primary endpoint, 28-day mortality, was similar with tifacogin and placebo, but the rate of bleeding was significantly higher with tifacogin.

NAPc2
Recombinant NAPc2 is a polypeptide originally isolated from the canine hookworm, *Ancylostoma caninum*, which is expressed in yeast. NAPc2 binds to a non-catalytic site on factor X or factor Xa. Once bound to factor Xa, the NAPc2/factor Xa complex inhibits tissue factor-bound factor VIIa. Because it binds factor X with high affinity, NAPc2 has a half-life of approximately 50 hours after subcutaneous injection. Consequently, the drug can be given on alternate days.

After promising results in an initial phase II clinical trial in venous thromboprophylaxis, the drug has been studied in phase II trials with arterial thrombosis and is currently being evaluated in PCI patients.

Factor VIIai
Inactivated factor VIIa (factor VIIai) competes with Factor VIIa for tissue factor binding, thereby modulating initiation of coagulation by the factor VIIa/tissue factor complex. Factor VIIai has been evaluated in a small study of patients undergoing elective percutaneous coronary interventions. The results were not sufficiently promising to continue its development for treatment of arterial thrombosis.

Factor IXa Inhibitors
Both parenteral and oral factor IXa inhibitors are under development. The parenteral factor IXa inhibitor is an RNA aptamer (RB006) that binds factor IXa with high affinity. RB006 can be neutralized rapidly by a complementary oligonucleotide (designated RB007). This drug–antidote pair is being developed for use in cardiopulmonary bypass surgery. An orally active, direct factor IXa inhibitor has also been developed.

Factor Xa Inhibitors

New factor Xa inhibitors include agents that block factor Xa indirectly or directly. Direct factor Xa inhibitors bind to the active site of factor Xa and inhibit both free and platelet-bound factor Xa. In contrast, indirect inhibitors act by catalyzing factor Xa inhibition by antithrombin, and have limited capacity to inhibit factor Xa incorporated into the prothrombinase complex.

Indirect Factor Xa Inhibitor

The prototype of the new indirect factor Xa inhibitors is fondaparinux. The newer indirect factor Xa inhibitors are designated idraparinux, SSR126517E, and SR123781A.

Idraparinux

Idraparinux, a hypermethylated derivative of fondaparinux, binds antithrombin with such high affinity that its plasma half-life of 80 hours is similar to that of antithrombin. It is given subcutaneously on a once-weekly basis. The anticoagulant has been evaluated in several phase III trials using a dose of 2.5 mg.

Idraparinux has been compared to conventional therapy with UFH or LMWH followed by a vitamin K antagonist in two separate phase III trials in deep vein thrombosis (DVT) and pulmonary embolism (PE). In the DVT trial, the rate of recurrent VTE at 3 months was similar in the idraparinux and conventionally-treated groups, but clinically relevant bleeds were less common with idraparinux. In the PE trial, idraparinux was less effective than conventional therapy at 3 months. Idraparinux has also been evaluated in patients who had completed 6 months of initial treatment of DVT or PE. Compared with placebo, idraparinux produced a 72.9% relative reduction in the risk of recurrent VTE ($p = .002$), but major bleeding occurred in 3.7% of those given idraparinux and included three fatal intracranial bleeds. In contrast, there were no major bleeds in the placebo group. Based on these data, it is unlikely that idraparinux will be developed further.

SSR12517E

A biotinylated form of idraparinux, SSR12517E exhibits the same pharmacokinetic and pharmacodynamic profile as idraparinux. The only difference is that the anticoagulant activity of SSR12517E can be rapidly neutralized by intravenous administration of avidin. SSR12517E is now undergoing phase III evaluation in patients with symptomatic PE with or without evidence of DVT.

SR123781A

SR123781A is a synthetic hexadecasaccharide composed of the antithrombin-binding synthetic pentasaccharide plus a thrombin binding sulfated tetrasaccharide joined together by a central nonsulfated heptasaccharide. SR123781A binds antithrombin with high affinity and, like heparin, catalyzes the inhibition of both factor Xa and thrombin. Unlike heparin, SR123781A does not bind PF4 or fibrin. SR123781A is administered subcutaneously. The drug is primarily cleared by the kidneys where it is excreted intact. SR123781A is currently undergoing phase II evaluation for prophylaxis in patients undergoing knee arthroplasty.

Direct Factor Xa Inhibitors

Direct factor Xa inhibitors include parenteral agents, DX9065a and otamixaban, as well as several orally active drugs. All of the direct factor Xa inhibitors are small molecules that reversibly block the active site of factor Xa.

DX-9065a

A synthetic nonpeptidic direct FXa inhibitor, DX9065a is administered parenterally. DX9065a was evaluated in patients with ACS but has not undergone further clinical evaluation.

Otamixaban

A noncompetitive inhibitor of FXa, this agent is administered intravenously and has a half-life of 2 to 3 hours. A phase II trial comparing otamixaban with heparin in patients with non–ST-elevation MI and planned early invasive strategy is under way.

Oral Factor Xa Inhibitors

Apixaban

Apixaban, a nonpeptide, has high oral bioavailability and a half-life of about 12 hours. Apixaban is cleared through both the fecal and renal route, with renal elimination accounting for about 25% of drug clearance.

Based on the promising results in a phase II trial in patients undergoing knee replacement surgery, a dose of 2.5 mg twice daily will be compared with enoxaparin in two phase III trials in patients undergoing knee replacement surgery and in one trial in patients undergoing hip replacement surgery. This dose will also be evaluated for thromboprophylaxis in medical patients. Phase II trials of apixaban for treatment of VTE, for secondary prevention in ACS patients, and for thromboprophylaxis in cancer patients are ongoing.

Rivaroxaban

Rivaroxaban is an oxazolidone derivative with oral bioavailability of 80% and a half-life of about 9 hours. It is cleared by the kidneys and the gut. Rivaroxaban has been evaluated for thromboprophylaxis in patients undergoing knee or hip arthroplasty in a series of phase II trials in enoxaparin-treated controls. There was no dose response in efficacy, but bleeding increased with dose. Overall, the results were promising and led to the selection of a 10 mg once-daily dose for future studies in major orthopedic surgery.

In a phase III clinical trial Regulation of Coagulation in Major Orthopaedic Surgery (RECORD)-3, rivaroxaban was compared with subcutaneous enoxaparin in 2,531 patients undergoing knee replacement surgery. Both regimens were continued for 10 to 14 days. The primary efficacy endpoint, a composite of DVT, non-fatal PE, and all-cause mortality, occurred in 9.6% of patients receiving rivaroxaban and in 18.9% of those given enoxaparin [a relative risk reduction of a 49%; ($p < .001$)]. Major venous thromboembolism (VTE), a composite of proximal DVT, non-fatal PE, and VTE-related mortality, occurred in 1.0% of patients given rivaroxaban and in 2.6% of those treated with enoxaparin; ($p = .01$). Major bleeding rates were 0.6% and 0.5% in the rivaroxaban and enoxaparin-treated groups, respectively, whereas any bleeding occurred in 4.9% and 4.8%, respectively. Three other phase III orthopedic trials have been conducted with rivaroxaban. Two are completed, and the third is under way.

Rivaroxaban also has been evaluated for treatment of proximal DVT in 2 phase II dose-ranging studies. The results were promising in terms of both efficacy and safety. Phase III studies evaluating rivaroxaban for treatment of VTE and for stroke prevention in atrial fibrillation are under way. A 20 mg once-daily dose of rivaroxaban is being evaluated for these indications.

LY-517717

LY-517717 has an oral bioavailability of 25 to 82% and a half-life of about 25 hours, allowing once-daily administration. LY-517717 has been evaluated in a phase II non-inferiority study in patients undergoing hip or knee arthroplasty. Additional studies are needed to determine the efficacy and safety of this agent.

YM 150

YM 150 is given once daily. It has been evaluated in a phase II study in patients undergoing elective hip arthroplasty. A second phase II trial in patients undergoing elective hip arthroplasty is ongoing.

DU-176b

DU-176b is currently undergoing phase II evaluation in hip arthroplasty patients.

PRT 054021

PRT 054021 has oral bioavailability of 47% and a half-life of 19 hours. It has been studied in a phase II trial in patients undergoing elective knee arthroplasty.

Factor Va Inhibitors

Drotrecogin Alfa (Activated)

Drotrecogin is a recombinant form of activated protein C and is licensed for treatment of patients with severe sepsis. Since approval, two additional clinical trials, one in adults with sepsis and a low risk of death, and the other in children with sepsis, were stopped prematurely due to lack of efficacy and the potential to cause harm because of bleeding.

ART-123

ART-123 a recombinant analog of the extracellular domain of thrombo-modulin, binds thrombin and converts it from a procoagulant enzyme into a potent activator of protein C. ART-123 has nearly 100% bioavailability after subcutaneous administration and a half-life of 2 to 3 days. It has been evaluated in a phase IIa dose-ranging study in patients undergoing elective hip arthroplasty. Plans for further development of this agent are uncertain.

Thrombin Inhibitors

Three parenteral direct thrombin inhibitors (hirudin, argatroban, and bivalirudin) have been licensed in North America for limited indications. Two new parenteral direct thrombin inhibitors and one new oral thrombin inhibitor are currently undergoing phase II evaluation.

Flovagatran

Flovagatran is a reversible, synthetic, active site–directed small molecule. The drug has a short half-life and is cleared via an extra-renal mechanism. Flovagatran is being investigated as an alternative to heparin during hemodialysis in patients with end-stage renal disease who have antibodies to the heparin/PF4 complex.

Pegmusirudin

Pegmusirudin is a hirudin derivative, chemically modified to prolong its half-life to about 12 hours. Like hirudin, pegmusirudin is cleared by the kidneys. The drug is undergoing phase II evaluation in patients with end-stage renal disease who are receiving routine hemodialysis.

Dabigatran Etexilate

Dabigatran etexilate has been evaluated for thromboprophylaxis in patients undergoing hip or knee arthroplasty and for prevention of stroke in patients with atrial fibrillation in phase II trials and in a phase III trial.

The phase III trial was a randomized trial of 2,076 patients that compared two doses of dabigatran and enoxaparin in patients undergoing knee arthroplasty. The incidence of the primary endpoint, a composite of total VTE and all-cause mortality, was similar in the three groups, as was the incidence of bleeding. Levels of alanine transaminase greater than three times the upper limit of normal were observed in 3.7% and 2.8% of patients receiving 150 and 220 mg of dabigatran etexilate, respectively, compared with 4.0% of those given enoxaparin.

Dabigatran etexilate has also been evaluated in two other phase III orthopedic trials. The RE-NOVATE trial randomized 3,494 patients undergoing hip replacement surgery to oral dabigatran etexilate or subcutaneous enoxaparin for an average of 33 days. The primary efficacy endpoint, a composite of DVT, non-fatal PE, and all-cause mortality, occurred in 8.6% and 6.0% of patients given dabigatran etexilate at 150 or 220 mg, respectively, and in 6.7% of those treated with enoxaparin. Major bleeding was similar in all three groups.

In the North American RE-MOBILIZE trial, patients undergoing knee replacement surgery were randomized to oral dabigatran etexilate or subcutaneous enoxaparin (30 mg twice daily, starting 12 to 24 hours after surgery) for 10 to 14 days. The primary efficacy endpoint, a composite of DVT, non-fatal PE, and all-cause mortality, occurred in 33.7% and 31.1% of patients treated with dabigatran at 150 or 220 mg, respectively, and in 25.3% of those given enoxaparin. Major bleeding occurred in 0.6% of patients treated with either dose of dabigatran and in 1.4% of those given enoxaparin, differences that were not statistically significant. Unlike the other two phase III trials, in which dabigatran showed non-inferiority to enoxaparin, dabigatran was inferior to enoxaparin in the RE-MOBILIZE trial. It has been speculated that this difference in relative efficacy may reflect the higher dose enoxaparin regimen used as a comparator and/or the delayed start of dabigatran etexilate.

A phase II trial in 502 patients with atrial fibrillation compared a three-month course of treatment with three different doses of dabigatran etexilate or with warfarin. Using a factorial design, patients were also randomized to aspirin (81 or 325 mg daily) or to placebo. The cumulative frequency of elevations in alanine transaminase of greater than three times the upper limit of normal was 2% in patients receiving dabigatran etexilate for at least 12 months, compared with 1% in those given warfarin. Based on the results of this phase II study, the phase III RELY trial is comparing dabigatran etexilate doses of 110 or 150 mg twice daily with dose-adjusted warfarin for stroke prevention in 18,000 patients with nonvalvular atrial fibrillation. In addition, dabigatran etexilate also is undergoing phase III evaluation for treatment of VTE.

New Fibrinolytic Agents

New fibrinolytic strategies include the development of inhibitors of type 1 plasminogen activator (PAI-1), activated factor XIII (factor XIIIa), and the new fibrinolytic agents alfimeprase, BB10153, and desmoteplase. Of these, only the new fibrinolytic agents have been tested clinically.

Alfimeprase

Alfimeprase is a recombinant truncated form of fibrolase. Like fibrolase, alfimeprase directly degrades the alpha-chain of fibrin and fibrinogen. The systemic effects of alfimeprase are attenuated by its rapid inhibition by α_2-macroglobulin. To bypass circulating α_2-macroglobulin, alfimeprase must be administered directly into the thrombus. Clinical trials of alfimeprase have focused on catheter-directed lysis of peripheral arterial occlusions or on local delivery to restore flow in indwelling catheters blocked by thrombus. Phase III studies with alfimeprase for these indications have been halted, at least temporarily, because key efficacy endpoints were not met. The full results of these trials have not yet been published.

BB10153

BB10153 is a variant form of plasminogen, in which the plasminogen activator cleavage site is replaced with a thrombin cleavage site. BB10153 binds to fibrin where it is converted to plasmin by fibrin-bound thrombin. After intravenous injection, BB10153 has a half-life of about 4.4 hours in humans. A phase II dose-escalation study in 50 patients with acute MI, produced promising results. BB10153 is currently undergoing evaluation for treatment of acute ischemic stroke and peripheral arterial occlusion.

Desmoteplase

Desmoteplase is a recombinant analog of the full-length plasminogen activator isolated from the saliva of the vampire bat. It has over 70% homology to tissue plasminogen activator (t-PA) and has greater fibrin specificity than t-PA. Desmoteplase is currently undergoing phase III evaluation for treatment of patients with acute ischemic stroke.

6 HEMORRHAGIC COMPLICATIONS OF ANTICOAGULANT AND THROMBOLYTIC TREATMENT

Bleeding is the major complication of antithrombotic and fibrinolytic therapy. In general, anticoagulant-induced bleeding is dose-related, although with vitamin K antagonists (VKAs) the direct relationship is with the intensity of the effect as reflected in the international normalized ratio (INR).

HEPARIN, LOW-MOLECULAR-WEIGHT HEPARIN, AND FONDAPARINUX

The risk of bleeding associated with intravenous unfractionated heparin (UFH) is dose-related, but the association between the level of the activated partial thromboplastin time (APTT) and bleeding is inconsistent. A relationship between bleeding and the APTT was not found in moderate-sized trials in of venous thrombosis, but was found in much larger studies in acute coronary syndrome patients.

Comorbid conditions, particularly recent surgery or trauma or recent stroke, are important risk factors for heparin-induced bleeding. Aspirin increases the risk of heparin-associated bleeding, as does the concomitant use of thrombolytic therapy or glycoprotein (GP) IIb-IIIa antagonists. Renal failure and patient age and sex have also been reported to be risk factors for heparin-induced bleeding.

When used postoperatively for prophylaxis against venous thromboembolism (VTE) (also called venous thromboembolic disease, venous thrombembolic event, or pulmonary embolism [PE]), the risk of bleeding with fondaparinux is inversely related to the timing of the first injection. Treatment with fondaparinux at a dose of 2.5 mg/d is associated with less bleeding than a therapeutic dose of low-molecular-weight heparin (LMWH) in patients with acute coronary syndrome (ACS), but in patients with VTE, a 7.5 mg/d dose of fondaparinux carried a similar risk of bleeding, as did therapeutic doses of UFH or LMWH.

Differences in the risk of bleeding among UFH, LMWH, and fondaparinux have been reported in clinical trials, but these differences may be related to the different intensities of the anticoagulant effect achieved, rather than to the intrinsic properties of the three classes of anticoagulants.

VITAMIN K ANTAGONISTS

The major determinants of VKA-induced bleeding are the intensity of the anticoagulant effect, underlying patient characteristics, concomitant use of drugs that interfere with hemostasis, and the length of therapy. A targeted INR of 2.5 (range: 2.0 to 3.0), is associated with a lower risk of bleeding than an INR > 3.0. The risk of bleeding increases dramatically with INR > 4.0–5.0. It is noteworthy, however, that even low-intensity warfarin is associated with an excess of major bleeding compared to placebo.

The risk of major bleeding during warfarin therapy is increased by patient age (particularly over 75) and a history of prior bleeding. Other patient-related factors include hypertension (treated and untreated) and cerebrovascular disease (both for intracranial bleeding), serious heart disease, diabetes, renal insufficiency, alcoholism, and liver disease.

Polymorphism of the cytochrome P450 CYP2C9 enzyme (the CYP2C9*2 and CYP2C9*3 variants) are associated with an increase in the risk of bleeding, presumably because of excessive dosing in patients who are slow metabolizers of VKAs. Patients with DVT have a higher rate of bleeding during the first three months of treatment than during subsequent long-term therapy.

The concomitant use of drugs that either impair platelet function or alter the pharmacokinetics of VKAs also increase the risk of bleeding.

DIRECT THROMBIN INHIBITORS

The irreversible direct thrombin inhibitor (DTI) hirudin is associated with a higher risk of bleeding than UFH in patients with ST-elevation myocardial infarction. In patients with unstable angina, bivalirudin or the low-molecular direct thrombin inhibitors appear to be safer than UFH.

THROMBOLYTIC THERAPY

Thrombolytic therapy increases the risk of major bleeding 1.5- to three-fold in patients with acute VTE, ischemic stroke, or ST-elevation myocardial infarction.

Advanced age, low body weight, prior cerebrovascular disease or hypertension, and randomization to tissue plasminogen activator (t-PA) (as opposed to streptokinase) have been reported as independent predictors of intracranial hemorrhage (ICH). In some studies female sex was also a risk factor for bleeding, probably because of lower body weight. Alteplase (t-PA) is associated with a higher risk of ICH than streptokinase.

ANTIPLATELET DRUGS

The risk of bleeding with single antiplatelet agents is lower than the risk with VKA. The risk of bleeding with aspirin is similar to the risk with clopidogrel. The combination of aspirin and clopidogrel is associated with more bleeding than either drug alone. The addition of aspirin to VKA increases the risk of bleeding over VKA alone. In contrast, the addition of dipyridamole to aspirin does not appear to increase the baseline rate of bleeding over that observed with aspirin alone. When aspirin is used in combination with either clopidogrel or VKA, the risk of bleeding is higher with high- versus low-dose aspirin.

7 PERIOPERATIVE MANAGEMENT OF ANTITHROMBOTIC THERAPY

This new chapter addresses the perioperative management of patients who are receiving vitamin K antagonists (VKAs) or antiplatelet drugs and require an elective or emergency surgical procedure. Most studies assessing perioperative management strategies have been observational, therefore, definitive recommendations cannot be made for most situations.

Three approaches can be used when managing patients receiving a VKA who require an invasive procedure. These are (1) stop anticoagulant therapy so the effect is no longer evident at the time of the procedure; (2) stop anticoagulant therapy before the procedure, but cover the patient with preoperative bridging with heparin of low-molecular-weight heparin (LMWH); and (3) continue warfarin therapy at a regular or lower intensity until the day before the procedure. In all these circumstances, postoperative bridging is introduced when indicated. Bridging, preoperatively and/or postoperatively, limits the duration that the patient is unprotected while not receiving VKA, but may increase the risk of bleeding. Preoperative bridging has minimal effects on bleeding risk, whereas postoperative bridging has the potential to increase postoperative bleeding.

Decisions about discontinuing routine antithrombotic therapy and use of bridging are based on patients' risks for bleeding with therapy and risks of thrombosis if therapy is temporarily discontinued.

RISK OF BLEEDING WITH ANTITHROMBOTIC THERAPY

In addition to systemic risk factors, certain operative procedures are associated with a high risk of bleeding. These are:

- coronary artery bypass or heart valve replacement surgery
- intracranial or spinal surgery
- aortic aneurysm repair, peripheral artery bypass, and other major vascular surgery

- major orthopedic surgery, such as hip or knee replacement
- reconstructive plastic surgery
- extensive cancer surgery
- prostate and bladder surgery
- resection of colonic polyps, especially sessile polyps > 2 cm in diameter
- biopsy of the prostate or kidney
- cardiac pacemaker or defibrillator implantation

In patients classified as high risk for stroke or thromboembolism, the need to prevent a thromboembolic event with bridging therapy will often override the bleeding risk. In patients classified as moderate risk for thromboembolism, the decision to use bridging therapy will depend on an individual risk assessment. In patients at low risk for thromboembolism, bridging therapy is usually avoided and, if used, limited to the preoperative period.

GENERAL PRINCIPLES UNDERLYING TIMING DECISIONS WITH PERIOPERATIVE ANTITHROMBOTICS

If the intent is to eliminate any effect of antithrombotic therapy at the time of the invasive procedure, warfarin should be stopped about 5 days preoperatively, and aspirin and clopidogrel should be stopped 7 to 10 days preoperatively.

The risk of bleeding with postoperative anticoagulant therapy increases with the dose of anticoagulant (eg, therapeutic dose > low dose) and the proximity to surgery.

For perioperative anticoagulants, there is evidence that low-dose LMWH or unfractionated heparin (UFH) is effective in preventing VTE, but there is no evidence that low-dose treatment is effective in preventing arterial thromboembolism.

When resuming antithrombotic therapy postoperatively, a substantial antithrombotic effect is observed within 2 to 3 days of starting warfarin, within minutes of starting aspirin [acetylsalicylic acid (ASA)], and within days of starting a maintenance dose of clopidogrel.

The three main indications for long-term oral anticoagulants are mechanical heart valve, chronic atrial fibrillation, and VTE.

Prosthetic Heart Valves

The efficacy of UFH or LMWH in patients with prosthetic heart valves is unknown. Further, there are no reliable data of the risk of perioperative arterial thromboembolism in patients with a mechanical heart valve who have warfarin stopped before surgery without bridging anticoagulation.

Although prospective cohort studies (in which bridging with therapeutic-dose LMWH regimens was used) reported a pooled risk for perioperative arterial thromboembolism of 0.83% (95% CI: 0.43 to 1.5), the interpretation of this pooled risk rate is uncertain.

Chronic Arial Fibrillation

The efficacy of UFH or LMWH in atrial fibrillation (AF) is unknown because randomized trials have not been performed comparing bridging with no bridging in AF patients. In studies of warfarin discontinuation without bridging, the reported risk for arterial thromboembolism in the perioperative period was about 1%. Although this rate is slightly higher than the 0.57% rate reported from prospective cohort studies that using bridging with low-dose and therapeutic-dose LMWH regimens, because of their indirectness, such comparisons are unreliable.

Patients with Prior Venous Thromboembolism

Low-dose UFH or LMWH is effective in preventing postoperative VTE. It is reasonable to assume, therefore, that prophylaxis would also be effective in patients with a history of VTE who require surgery.

ANTIPLATELET THERAPY

Patients at high risk for cardiovascular events should be considered for continuation of antiplatelet therapy perioperatively. High-risk patients are those who have had placement of a bare-metal or drug-eluting coronary stent, and those who have suffered a myocardial infarction within the prior 3 months.

Coronary Artery Bypass Graft Surgery

There is evidence that preoperative clopidogrel increases the risk of bleeding associated with coronary artery bypass graft (CABG) surgery. There is also evidence that preoperative aspirin increases the risk of bleeding in CABG patients. On the other hand, there is evidence that preoperative aspirin may reduce the risk of postoperative mortality, and that clopidogrel reduces the risk of stent thrombosis. If aspirin therapy has been interrupted before surgery, it should be administered early after surgery, preferably within 6 hours after surgery.

Percutaneous Coronary Interventions

Patients who are receiving aspirin and clopidogrel before percutaneous coronary intervention (PCI) should continue taking these drugs in the periprocedural period.

MANAGEMENT OF URGENT SURGICAL OR OTHER INVASIVE PROCEDURES

Anticoagulants

Patients who require rapid (within 12 hours) reversal of the anticoagulant effects of VKAs because of an urgent surgical or other invasive procedure can be treated in a number of ways. These include fresh-frozen plasma, prothrombin concentrates, and recombinant factor VIIa. In addition, such patients should receive vitamin K, because the effects of warfarin persist after replacement therapy.

Antiplatelet Drugs

Patients who require urgent surgery and who have a major bleed in the perioperative period can be treated with platelet transfusion.

RECOMMENDATIONS

Perioperative Management of Patients Who Are Receiving Vitamin K Antagonists

1. In patients who require temporary interruption of VKA before surgery or a procedure, and who require normalization of the INR for the surgery or procedure, we recommend stopping VKAs approximately 5 days before surgery over stopping VKAs within a shorter time interval before surgery to allow adequate time for the INR to normalize **(Grade 1B)**.

2. In patients who have had temporary interruption of VKA before surgery or a procedure, we recommend resuming VKAs approximately 12 to 24 hours (the evening of, or the next morning) after surgery and when there is adequate hemostasis, rather than resumption of VKAs closer to surgery **(Grade 1C)**.

3. In patients who require temporary interruption of VKA before surgery or a procedure and whose INR is still elevated (ie, ≥ 1.5) 1 to 2 days before surgery, we suggest administering low-dose (ie, 1 to 2 mg) oral vitamin K to normalize the INR instead of not administering vitamin K **(Grade 2C)**.

4. In patients with a mechanical heart valve or atrial fibrillation or VTE at high risk for thromboembolism, we recommend bridging anticoagulation with therapeutic-dose subcutaneous (SC) LMWH or intravenous (IV) UFH over no bridging during temporary interruption of VKA therapy **(Grade 1C)**; we suggest therapeutic-dose SC LMWH over IV UFH **(Grade 2C)**. In patients with a mechanical heart valve or atrial fibrillation or VTE at moderate risk for thromboembolism, we suggest

bridging anticoagulation with therapeutic-dose SC LMWH, therapeutic-dose IV UFH, or low-dose SC LMWH over no bridging during temporary interruption of VKA therapy **(Grade 2C)**; we suggest therapeutic-dose SC LMWH over other bridging options **(Grade 2C)**. In patients with a mechanical heart valve or atrial fibrillation or VTE at low risk for thromboembolism, we suggest low-dose SC LMWH or no bridging over bridging with therapeutic-dose SC LMWH or IV UFH **(Grade 2C)**.

Perioperative Management of Patients Who Are Receiving Bridging Anticoagulation

1. In patients who require temporary interruption of VKAs and who are to receive bridging anticoagulation, from a cost containment perspective, we recommend the use of SC LMWH administered in an outpatient setting (where feasible) instead of inpatient administration of IV UFH **(Grade 1C)**.

2. In patients who are receiving bridging anticoagulation with therapeutic-dose SC LMWH, we recommend administering the last dose of LMWH 24 hours before surgery or procedure rather than administering LMWH closer to surgery **(Grade 1C)**; for the last preoperative dose of LMWH, we recommend administering approximately half the total daily dose instead of 100% of the total daily dose **(Grade 1C)**. In patients who are receiving bridging anticoagulation with therapeutic-dose IV UFH, we recommend stopping UFH approximately 4 hours before surgery over stopping UFH closer to surgery **(Grade 1C)**.

3. In patients undergoing a minor surgical or other invasive procedure and who are receiving bridging anticoagulation with therapeutic-dose LMWH, we recommend resuming this regimen approximately 24 hours after (eg, the day after) the procedure when there is adequate hemostasis over a shorter (eg, < 12 hours) time interval **(Grade 1C)**. In patients undergoing major surgery or a high–bleeding-risk surgery/procedure and for whom postoperative therapeutic-dose LMWH/UFH is planned, we recommend either delaying the initiation of therapeutic-dose LMWH/UFH for 48 to 72 hours after surgery when hemostasis is secured, administering low-dose LMWH after surgery when hemostasis is secured, or completely avoiding LMWH or UFH after surgery rather than the administration of therapeutic-dose LMWH/UFH in close proximity to surgery **(Grade 1C)**. We recommend consideration of the anticipated bleeding risk and of the adequacy of postoperative hemostasis in individual patients in order to determine the timing of LMWH or UFH resumption after surgery instead of resuming LMWH or UFH at a fixed time after surgery in all patients **(Grade 1C)**.

4. In patients who are receiving bridging anticoagulation with LMWH, we suggest that the routine use of anti-factor Xa levels to monitor the anticoagulant effect of LMWHs should not be used **(Grade 2C).**

Perioperative Management of Patients Who Are Receiving Antiplatelet Therapy

1. In patients who require temporary interruption of aspirin- or clopido-grel-containing drugs before their surgery or procedure, we suggest stopping this treatment 7 to 10 days before the procedure over stopping this treatment closer to surgery **(Grade 2C)**.
2. In patients who have had temporary interruption of aspirin or clopidogrel therapy because of surgery or a procedure, we suggest resuming aspirin or clopidogrel approximately 24 hours (or the next morning) after surgery when there is adequate hemostasis instead of resuming aspirin or clopidogrel closer to surgery **(Grade 2C)**.
3. In patients who are receiving antiplatelet drugs, we suggest against the routine use of platelet function assays to monitor the antithrombotic effect of aspirin or clopidogrel **(Grade 2C)**.
4. For patients who are not at high risk for cardiac events, we recommend interruption of antiplatelet drugs **(Grade 1C)**. For patients at high risk of cardiac events (exclusive of coronary stents) scheduled for non-cardiac surgery, we suggest continuing aspirin up to and beyond the time of surgery **(Grade 2C)**; if patients are receiving clopidogrel, we suggest interrupting clopidogrel at least 5 days and, preferably, within 10 days prior to surgery **(Grade 2C)**. In patients scheduled for CABG, we recommend continuing aspirin up to and beyond the time of CABG **(Grade 1C)**; if aspirin is interrupted, we recommend it be reinitiated between 6 hours and 48 hours after CABG **(Grade 1C)**. In patients scheduled for CABG, we recommend interrupting clopidogrel at least 5 days and, preferably, 10 days prior to surgery **(Grade 1C)**. In patients scheduled for PCI, we suggest continuing aspirin up to and beyond the time of the procedure; if clopidogrel is interrupted prior to PCI, we suggest resuming clopidogrel after PCI with a loading dose of 300 to 600 mg **(Grade 2C)**.
5. In patients with a bare-metal coronary stent who require surgery within 6 weeks of stent placement, we recommend continuing aspirin and clopidogrel in the perioperative period **(Grade 1C)**. In patients with a drug-eluting coronary stent who require surgery within 12 months of stent placement, we recommend continuing aspirin and clopidogrel in the perioperative period **(Grade 1C)**. In patients with a coronary stent who have interruption of antiplatelet therapy before surgery, we suggest against the routine use of bridging therapy with

UFH, LMWH, direct thrombin inhibitors, or glycoprotein IIb/IIIa inhibitors **(Grade 2C)**.

Perioperative Management of Antithrombotic Therapy in Patients Who Require Dental, Dermatologic, or Ophthalmologic Procedures

1. In patients who are undergoing minor dental procedures and who are receiving VKAs, we recommend continuing VKAs around the time of the procedure and co-administering an oral prohemostatic agent **(Grade 1B)**. In patients who are undergoing minor dental procedures and who are receiving aspirin, we recommend continuing aspirin around the time of the procedure **(Grade 1C)**. In patients who are undergoing minor dental procedures and are receiving clopidogrel, please refer to the recommendations outlined above.

2. In patients who are undergoing minor dermatologic procedures and who are receiving VKAs, we recommend continuing VKAs around the time of the procedure **(Grade 1C)**. In patients who are undergoing minor dermatologic procedures and who are receiving aspirin, we recommend continuing aspirin around the time of the procedure **(Grade 1C)**. In patients who are undergoing minor dermatologic procedures and who are receiving clopidogrel, please refer to the recommendations outlined above.

3. In patients who are undergoing cataract removal and who are receiving VKAs, we recommend continuing VKAs around the time of the procedure **(Grade 1C)**. In patients who are undergoing cataract removal and who are receiving aspirin, we recommend continuing aspirin around the time of the procedure **(Grade 1C)**. In patients who are undergoing cataract removal and who are receiving clopidogrel, please refer to the recommendations outlined above.

Perioperative Management of Antithrombotic Therapy in Patients Who Require Urgent Surgical or Other Invasive Procedures

1. In patients who are receiving VKAs and who require reversal of the anticoagulant effect for an urgent surgical or other invasive procedure, we recommend treatment with low-dose (2.5 to 5.0 mg) intravenous or oral vitamin K **(Grade 1C)**. For more immediate reversal of the anticoagulant effect, we suggest treatment with fresh-frozen plasma or another prothrombin concentrate in addition to low-dose intravenous or oral vitamin K **(Grade 2C)**.

2. For patients receiving aspirin, clopidogrel, or both, and who are undergoing surgery, and who have excessive or life-threatening perioperative

bleeding, we suggest transfusion of platelets or administration of other prohemostatic agents in patients **(Grade 2C)**.

8 TREATMENT AND PREVENTION OF HEPARIN-INDUCED THROMBOCYTOPENIA: CLINICAL FEATURES AND DIAGNOSIS

Heparin-induced thrombocytopenia (HIT) is an antibody-mediated adverse effect of heparin. It is important because of its strong association with venous and arterial thrombosis. The thrombotic tendency in HIT is caused by immune-mediated platelet activation. The thrombotic manifestations include venous and arterial thrombosis.

The frequency of HIT among patients exposed to heparin is higher with heparin than low-molecular-weight heparin (LMWH), is higher in surgical patients than medical patients, and is very low in pregnancy. These differences in risk influence the required frequency of platelet count monitoring in patients receiving heparin.

A diagnosis of HIT should be suspected if the platelet count falls by 50% or more of the baseline count (the count preceding such a fall) during 5 to 10 days of heparin treatment. It should also be suspected if a thrombotic complication or heparin-induced skin lesions occur during or soon after heparin treatment or if an acute systemic reaction occurs following an intravenous bolus dose of heparin.

A diagnosis of HIT is made when any of the following events occur in association with the presence of HIT antibodies detected by in vitro assays: (1) an otherwise unexplained platelet count fall of at least 50%; (2) venous or arterial thrombosis (even in the absence of a 50% fall in platelet count), (3) skin lesions at heparin injection sites (even in the absence of a 50% fall in platelet count), or (4) acute systemic (anaphylactoid) reactions that occur after administration of an intravenous bolus of heparin. A positive platelet activation assay is much more specific for clinical HIT than a positive platelet factor 4 (PF4)-dependent immunoassay. In about 25% of HIT patients, a thrombotic event during heparin treatment *precedes* the subsequent HIT-associated platelet count fall.

Although, in HIT patients, the platelet count usually begins to fall 5 to 10 days after commencing heparin, there are also other patterns of platelet count fall. Thus, in about 25 to 30% of patients, the platelet count falls abruptly upon beginning heparin; typically, these patients have recently been exposed to heparin and have HIT antibodies. In a much smaller percentage of patients, the onset of thrombocytopenia begins several days after heparin has been stopped. The diagnosis of HIT is confirmed by detecting HIT antibodies on serologic testing.

TREATMENT

When HIT is suspected, heparin should be discontinued, and if anticoagulant therapy is indicated, heparin should be replaced with an anticoagulant that does not cross-react with HIT antibodies. Currently, there are four anticoagulants available that do not cross-react with HIT antibodies. Of these, three direct thrombin inhibitors, argatroban, lepirudin (hirudin), and bivalirudin, are approved for treatment of HIT in the United States [bivalirudin is approved only for patients undergoing percutaneous coronary intervention (PCI)]. Fondaparinux, an antithrombin-dependent factor Xa inhibitor, is being used off-label to a limited extent. A fifth agent, danaparoid, which exhibits minimal cross-reactivity with HIT antibodies, was recently withdrawn from the US and UK markets, but is approved for treatment and prevention of HIT-associated thrombosis in other counties.

The optimal management of HIT without thrombosis remains uncertain. Many such patients either have silent venous thrombosis or are at risk of developing venous thrombosis in the ensuing days. The use of vitamin K antagonists (without a thrombin inhibitor) to treat such patients should be avoided because it carries a risk of venous gangrene. If anticoagulation is indicated, an anticoagulant that does not react with HIT antibodies and that is of proven effectiveness should be used until the platelet count returns to normal levels, and the introduction of warfarin should be delayed until there has been substantial recovery of thrombocytopenia.

Most clinical experience for the treatment of HIT has been obtained with hirudin and argatroban. The choice between hirudin and argatroban is influenced by renal and hepatic status of the patient. Argatroban should be used in cases of renal failure, whereas hirudin should be selected in cases of liver disease. Most clinical experience in non-HIT patients undergoing PCI is with bivalirudin. Most clinical experience in deep vein thrombosis (DVT) prophylaxis, in VTE treatment, and in acute coronary syndrome (ACS) treatment in non-HIT patients has been obtained with fondaparinux, but fondaparinux is not approved for HIT. Platelet transfusions are not indicated for the prevention of bleeding in patients with acute HIT, because bleeding is very uncommon in HIT and it is possible that platelet transfusions could contribute to the risk of thrombotic events.

CARDIOPULMONARY BYPASS SURGERY

The appropriate method of anticoagulation of patients with a history of proven or suspected HIT who require cardiac bypass surgery is controversial. The risk of rapid-onset HIT with transient exposure to heparin during surgery is very low or negligible if the last exposure to heparin was greater than 100 days and/or if the patient does not have circulating HIT antibodies.

The use of an alternative anticoagulant during cardiopulmonary bypass surgery is problematic, both because of the limited experience with alternative anticoagulants in cardiac surgical patients and the difficulty in their reversal after surgery. Based on the scientific rationale and limited clinical data on the safety of heparin re-exposure, it is likely that intraoperative unfractionated heparin (UFH) exposure is safe, provided that HIT antibodies are absent and previous exposure to heparin was remote.

RECOMMENDATIONS

Recognition of HIT

1. For patients receiving heparin in whom the clinician considers the risk of HIT to be > 1.0%, we recommend platelet count monitoring over no platelet count monitoring **(Grade 1C)**. For patients receiving heparin who have an estimated risk of HIT of 0.1 to 1.0%, we suggest platelet count monitoring over no platelet count monitoring **(Grade 2C)**.

Platelet Count Monitoring of Patients Recently Treated With Heparin

1. For patients who are starting UFH or LMWH treatment and who have received UFH within the past 100 days, or those patients in whom exposure history is uncertain, we recommend obtaining a baseline platelet count and then a repeat platelet count within 24 hours of starting heparin over not obtaining a repeat platelet count **(Grade 1C)**.

Anaphylactoid Reactions Post-IV UFH Bolus

1. For patients in whom acute inflammatory, cardiorespiratory, neurologic, or other unusual symptoms and signs develop within 30 minutes following an intravenous (IV) UFH bolus, we recommend performing an immediate platelet count measurement, comparing this value to recent prior platelet counts, rather than not performing a platelet count **(Grade 1C)**.

Platelet Count Monitoring in Patients Receiving Therapeutic-Dose UFH

1. For patients who are receiving therapeutic-dose UFH, we suggest platelet count monitoring at least every 2 or 3 days from day 4 to day

14 (or until heparin is stopped, whichever occurs first) over less frequent platelet count monitoring **(Grade 2C)**.

Platelet Count Monitoring in Postoperative Patients Receiving UFH Antithrombotic Prophylaxis (Highest Risk Group for HIT)

1. For patients who are receiving postoperative antithrombotic prophylaxis with UFH, ie, the patient population at highest risk for HIT (HIT risk > 1%), we suggest platelet count monitoring at least every other day between postoperative days 4 to 14 (or until UFH is stopped, whichever occurs first) over less frequent platelet count monitoring **(Grade 2C)**.

Platelet Count Monitoring in Patients in Whom HIT Is Infrequent (0.1 to 1%)

1. For medical/obstetrical patients who are receiving prophylactic-dose UFH, postoperative patients receiving prophylactic-dose LMWH, postoperative patients receiving intravascular catheter UFH "flushes," or medical/obstetrical patients receiving LMWH after first receiving UFH (estimated HIT risk, 0.1 to 1%), we suggest platelet count monitoring at least every 2 or 3 days from day 4 to day 14 (or until heparin is stopped, whichever occurs first), when practical, over less frequent platelet count monitoring **(Grade 2C)**.

Platelet Count Monitoring When HIT Is Rare (< 0.1%): UFH and LMWH

1. For medical/obstetrical patients who are receiving only LMWH, or medical patients who are receiving only intravascular catheter UFH "flushes" (HIT risk < 0.1%), we suggest clinicians do not use routine platelet count monitoring **(Grade 2C)**.

Platelet Count Monitoring When HIT Is Rare (< 0.1%): Fondaparinux

1. For patients who are receiving fondaparinux thromboprophylaxis or treatment, we recommend that clinicians do not use routine platelet count monitoring **(Grade 1C)**.

Management of Patients in Whom Platelet Counts Are Not Monitored

1. In outpatients who will receive heparin prophylaxis or treatment, informed consent should include HIT and its typical sequelae (new

thrombosis, skin lesions), and the patient should be advised to seek medical advice if these events occur **(Grade 2C)**.

Screening for Subclinical HIT Antibody Seroconversion

1. In patients who receive heparin or in whom heparin treatment is planned (eg, for cardiac or vascular surgery), we recommend against routine HIT antibody testing in the absence of thrombocytopenia, thrombosis, heparin-induced skin lesions, or other signs pointing to a potential diagnosis of HIT **(Grade 1C)**.

When Should HIT Be Suspected?

1. For patients who are receiving heparin or who have received heparin within the previous 2 weeks, we recommend investigating for a diagnosis of HIT if the platelet count falls by 50% or more, and/or a thrombotic event occurs, between days 5 and 14 (inclusive) following initiation of heparin, even if the patient is no longer receiving heparin therapy when thrombosis or thrombocytopenia has occurred **(Grade 1C)**.

Special Situation: Anticoagulant Prophylaxis and Platelet Count Monitoring After Cardiac Surgery

1. For postoperative cardiac surgery patients, we recommend investigating for HIT antibodies if the platelet count falls by 50% or more, and/or a thrombotic event occurs, between postoperative days 5 and 14 (inclusive; day of cardiac surgery = day 0) **(Grade 1C)**.

Treatment of HIT

Non-heparin Anticoagulants for Treating HIT (With or Without Thrombosis)

1. For patients with strongly suspected (or confirmed) HIT, whether or not complicated by thrombosis, we recommend use of an alternative, non-heparin anticoagulant [danaparoid **(Grade 1B)**, lepirudin **(Grade 1C)**, argatroban **(Grade 1C)**, fondaparinux **(Grade 2C)**, bivalirudin **(Grade 2C)**] over the further use of UFH or LMWH therapy or initiation/continuation of vitamin K antagonist (VKA) **(Grade 1B)**.

2. For patients receiving lepirudin, the initial lepirudin infusion rate should be no higher than 0.10 mg/kg/h (patients with creatinine < 90 μmol/L), with lower infusion rates for patients with higher serum creatinine levels (creatinine, 90 to 140 μmol/L: starting infusion rate, 0.05 mg/kg/h; creatinine, 140 to 400 μmol/L: starting infusion rate, 0.01 mg/kg/h; creatinine > 400 μmol/L: starting infusion rate, 0.005 mg/kg/h) **(Grade 1C)**. Furthermore, we recommend that the initial

IV bolus either be omitted or, in case of perceived life- or limb-threatening thrombosis, be given at a reduced dose (0.2 mg/kg) **(Grade 1C)**. Further, we recommend that activated partial thromboplastin time (APTT) monitoring be performed at 4-hour intervals until it is apparent that steady state within the normal range [1.5 to 2.5 times patient baseline (or mean laboratory) APTT] is achieved **(Grade 1C)**.

3. When argatroban is used to treat patients who have heart failure, multiple organ system failure, or severe anasarca or who are post cardiac surgery, we suggest beginning the initial infusion at a rate between 0.5 and 1.2 µg/kg/min, with subsequent adjustments using the APTT, rather than the usual recommended starting dose of 2.0 µg/kg/min **(Grade 2C)**.

4. When danaparoid is used to treat patients with strongly suspected (or confirmed) HIT, we recommend a therapeutic-dose regimen administered (at least initially) by the IV route rather than prophylactic-dose regimens or initial SC administration **(Grade 1B)**.

5. For patients with strongly suspected or confirmed HIT, whether or not there is clinical evidence of lower-limb DVT, we recommend routine ultrasonography of the lower-limb veins for investigation of DVT over not performing routine ultrasonography **(Grade 1C)**.

Vitamin K Antagonists

Management of Direct Thrombin Inhibitor–Vitamin K Antagonist Overlap

1. For patients with strongly suspected or confirmed HIT, we recommend against the use of VKA (coumarin) therapy until after the platelet count has substantially recovered (ie, usually to at least 150 × 10^9/L and, preferably, to a stable plateau) over starting VKA therapy at a lower platelet count **(Grade 1B)**. VKA therapy should be started only with low, maintenance doses (maximum, 5 mg of warfarin or 6 mg of phenprocoumon) rather than with higher initial doses **(Grade 1B)**, and there should be a minimum overlap of at least 5 days between non-heparin anticoagulation (eg, lepirudin, argatroban, danaparoid) and VKA therapy rather than a shorter overlap **(Grade 1B)**.

Reversal of VKA Anticoagulation

1. For patients receiving VKA at the time of diagnosis of HIT, we recommend use of vitamin K (10 mg orally or 5 to 10 mg IV) **(Grade 1C)**.

LMWH for HIT

1. For patients with strongly suspected HIT, whether or not complicated by thrombosis, we recommend against use of LMWH **(Grade 1B)**.

Prophylactic Platelet Transfusions for HIT

1. For patients with strongly suspected or confirmed HIT who do not have active bleeding, we suggest that prophylactic platelet transfusions not be given **(Grade 2C)**.

Special Patient Populations

Patients With Previous HIT Undergoing Cardiac or Vascular Surgery

1. For patients with a history of HIT who are HIT antibody negative and require cardiac surgery, we recommend the use of UFH over a non-heparin anticoagulant **(Grade 1B)**.
2. For patients with a history of HIT who are antibody positive by PF4-dependent ELISA assay but antibody negative by washed platelet activation assay, we recommend the use of UFH over a non-heparin anticoagulant **(Grade 2C)**.

Patients With Acute or Subacute HIT Undergoing Cardiac Surgery

1. For patients with acute HIT (thrombocytopenic, HIT antibody positive) who require cardiac surgery, we recommend one of the following alternative anticoagulant approaches (in descending order of preference):
   * delaying surgery (if possible) until HIT has resolved and antibodies are negative (then see recommendation 1 above) or weakly positive (then see recommendation 2 above) **(Grade 1B)**;
   * using bivalirudin for intraoperative anticoagulation during cardiopulmonary bypass (if techniques of cardiac surgery and anesthesiology have been adapted to the unique features of bivalirudin pharmacology) **(Grade 1B)** or during "off-pump" cardiac surgery **(Grade 1B)**;
   * using lepirudin for intraoperative anticoagulation [if Ecarin Clotting Time (ECT) is available and patient has normal renal function and is judged to be at low risk for postcardiac surgery renal dysfunction] **(Grade 2C)**;
   * using UFH plus the antiplatelet agent epoprostenol (if ECT monitoring is not available or renal insufficiency precludes lepirudin use) **(Grade 2C)**;

- using UFH plus the antiplatelet agent, tirofiban **(Grade 2C)**; or using danaparoid for intraoperative anticoagulation for "off-pump" coronary artery bypass surgery **(Grade 2C)** rather than performing the surgery with UFH when platelet-activating anti-PF4/heparin antibodies are known to be present in a patient with acute or recent HIT.

2. For patients with subacute HIT (platelet count recovery, but continuing HIT antibody positive), we recommend delaying surgery (if possible) until HIT antibodies (washed platelet activation assay) are negative, then using heparin (see recommendation 1 above) over using a non-heparin anticoagulant **(Grade 1C)**. If surgery cannot be delayed, we suggest the use of a non-heparin anticoagulant over the use of UFH **(Grade 2C)**.

Percutaneous Coronary Interventions

1. For patients with strongly suspected (or confirmed) acute HIT who require cardiac catheterization or PCI, we recommend a non-heparin anticoagulant [bivalirudin **(Grade 1B)**, argatroban **(Grade 1C)**, lepirudin **(Grade 1C)**, or danaparoid **(Grade 1C)**] over UFH or LMWH **(Grade 1B)**.

2. For patients with previous HIT (who are antibody negative) who require cardiac catheterization or PCI, we suggest use of a non-heparin anticoagulant over heparin or LMWH **(Grade 2C)**.

9 PREVENTION OF VENOUS THROMBOEMBOLISM

Pulmonary embolism (PE) is the most common cause of preventable death in hospitalized patients. Almost all hospitalized patients have at least one risk factor for VTE, and about 40% have three or more risk factors. Prophylaxis is highly effective in reducing the risk of deep vein thrombosis (DVT), PE, and fatal PE and should be used in most hospitalized patients. Various strategies improve adherence to evidence-based guidelines on the use of prophylaxis, including audit and feedback, automatic reminders, and the use of preprinted orders.

The important clinical risk factors for VTE include advanced age, general anesthesia, prolonged immobility or paralysis, previous VTE, cancer, duration of surgery, orthopedic surgery of lower limb leg, hip or pelvic fracture, major trauma, stroke, obesity, varicose veins, postoperative infection, and heart failure.

Venous thromboembolism can be prevented either by reducing venous stasis or by counteracting increased blood coagulability with anticoagulants.

REDUCING VENOUS STASIS

Mobilization alone does not provide adequate thromboprophylaxis for high-risk patients. Mechanical methods of prophylaxis, which include graduated compression stockings (GCS), intermittent pneumatic compression (IPC) devices, and the venous foot pump (VFP), increase venous outflow and/or reduce venous stasis. They have the advantage of being free of bleeding potential, but physical methods have been studied much less intensively than anticoagulant prophylaxis. In addition, because of problems with compliance and with optimal fitting, they are unlikely to be as effective in routine clinical practice as in clinical trials. Therefore mechanical prophylaxis is the preferred option only in patients at high risk for bleeding, but might also be considered in combination with anticoagulant prophylaxis in very-high-risk groups.

REDUCING BLOOD COAGULABILITY (ANTICOAGULANTS)

The anticoagulants that have been shown to be effective for prophylaxis are unfractionated heparin (UFH), low-molecular-weight heparin (LMWH), vitamin K antagonists (VKA), and fondaparinux. Renal clearance is the primary mode of elimination of LMWH and fondaparinux. Accordingly these drugs may accumulate and increase the risk of bleeding in patients with reduced renal function.

GENERAL SURGERY

Patients undergoing general surgery, gynecologic surgery, vascular surgery, and laparoscopic surgery can be classified into various risk categories. For those at low risk, prophylaxis is limited to early mobilization. Most patients undergoing outpatient surgery are at low risk for DVT. Active prophylaxis is indicated for all other risk categories. Low-dose heparin, external pneumatic compression, graduated compression stockings, LMWHs, fondaparinux and oral anticoagulants have all been shown to be effective in general surgery patients. Thromboprophylaxis using either low-dose heparin or LMWH (nadroparin) was shown to reduce mortality in two separate trials.

In high-risk general-surgery patients, higher doses of LMWH tend to provide greater protection than lower doses of the same LMWH, but higher doses increase the risk of bleeding. If an LMWH preparation is used for thromboprophylaxis, it should be administered in the doses recommended on the manufacturer's label.

ORTHOPEDIC SURGERY

For elective hip surgery patients, fondaparinux, LMWHs, and oral antico-agulants are most effective. Of these three methods, fondaparinux is more effective than LMWH; LMWH is more effective than warfarin or low-dose heparin; and warfarin is more effective than aspirin. For elective total knee replacement (TKR) patients, LMWH is more effective than low-dose heparin or warfarin, and fondaparinux is more effective than LMWH but at the cost of an increase in bleeding. For patients with hip fracture, fonda-parinux is most effective, and warfarin is more effective than aspirin; data on LMWH are relatively sparse in hip fracture patients.

Contemporary studies have shown that patients undergoing elective hip surgery or surgery for hip fracture remain at substantial risk of postop-erative thrombosis (detected by venography) despite the use of prophylaxis for 7 to 10 days postoperatively. The use of LMWH for up to 35 days post-operatively is effective in reducing the incidence of these late thrombi in elective hip surgery, and fondaparinux for 30 days is effective in reducing the incidence of late thrombosis in hip fracture patients. Warfarin is also effective as an extended prophylaxis in total hip replacement patients, but its use is associated with more bleeding than LMWH.

OTHER SURGERY

Both external pneumatic compression and LMWH are effective in pre-venting thrombosis in neurosurgery patients. If available, the first approach is probably preferred because it does not carry an increased risk of bleed-ing. For patients with spinal cord injury, LMWH appears to be effective, whereas low-dose heparin, intermittent pneumatic compression, and grad-uated compression stockings provide inadequate protection.

MEDICAL CONDITIONS

Over 50% of symptomatic thromboembolic events, and over 70% of fatal PE occur in nonsurgical patients. Therefore appropriate prophylaxis of medical inpatients is important. LMWH, low-dose heparin and fonda-parinux have all been shown to be effective methods of prophylaxis in medical patients.

The recommended methods of prophylaxis for low-, moderate- and high-risk categories are summarized in Table 1.

Table 9-1 Recommended Methods of Prophylaxis

Level of Risk	Suggested Prophylactic Options
Low Risk	
Minor surgery in mobile patients	No specific prophylaxis: early and
Medical patients who are fully mobile	aggressive ambulation
Moderate Risk	
Most general, open gynecologic or	LMWH (at recommended dose)
urologic surgical patients	or
Medical patients at bed rest or	Low-dose UFH (bid or tid)
who are sick	or
	Fondaparinux
Moderate VTE Risk +	Mechanical prophylaxis★
High Bleeding Risk	
High Risk	
Hip or knee arthroplasty, hip fracture	LMWH (at recommended doses)
surgery	or
Major trauma, spinal cord injury	Fondaparinux
	or
	Vitamin K antagonists (INR: 2.0 to 3.0)
High VTE Risk + Bleeding Risk	Mechanical prophylaxis★

★Mechanical prophylaxis includes intermittent pneumatic compression devices, or venous foot pump and /or graduated compression stockings. Consider switching to anticoagulant prophylaxis when bleeding risk decreases.
bid = twice daily; INR = international normalized ratio; LMWH = low-molecular-weight heparin; tid = three times a day; UFH = unfractionated heparin.

RECOMMENDATIONS

Hospital Thromboprophylaxis Policy

1. For every general hospital, we recommend that a formal, active strategy that addresses the prevention of VTE be developed **(Grade 1A)**.

2. We recommend that the local thromboprophylaxis strategy be in the form of a written, institution-wide thromboprophylaxis policy **(Grade 1C)**.

3. We recommend the use of strategies shown to increase thromboprophylaxis adherence, including the use of computer decision-support systems **(Grade 1A)**, preprinted orders **(Grade 1B)**, and periodic audit and feedback **(Grade 1C)**. Passive methods, such as distribution of educational materials or educational meetings, are not recom-

mended as sole strategies to increase adherence to thromboprophylaxis **(Grade 1B)**.

Mechanical Methods of Thromboprophylaxis

1. We recommend that mechanical methods of thromboprophylaxis be used primarily in patients at high risk of bleeding **(Grade 1A)**, or possibly as an adjunct to anticoagulant-based thromboprophylaxis **(Grade 2A)**.
2. For patients receiving mechanical methods of thromboprophylaxis, we recommend that careful attention be directed toward ensuring the proper use of, and optimal adherence with, these methods **(Grade 1A)**.

Aspirin as Thromboprophylaxis

1. We recommend *against* the use of aspirin alone as thromboprophylaxis against VTE for any patient group **(Grade 1A)**.

Anticoagulant Dosing

1. For each of the antithrombotic agents, we recommend that clinicians follow the manufacturers' suggested dosing guidelines **(Grade 1C)**.

Renal Impairment and Anticoagulant Dosing

1. We recommend that renal function be considered when making decisions about the use and/or dose of LMWH, fondaparinux, and other antithrombotic drugs that are cleared by the kidneys, particularly in elderly patients, patients with diabetes mellitus, and those at high risk for bleeding **(Grade 1A)**. Depending on the circumstances, we recommend one of the following options in this situation: avoiding the use of an anticoagulant that bioaccumulates in the presence of renal impairment, using a lower dose of the agent, or monitoring the drug level or its anticoagulant effect **(Grade 1B)**.

Antithrombotic Drugs and Neuraxial Anesthesia/Analgesia or Peripheral Nerve Blocks

1. For all patients undergoing neuraxial anesthesia or analgesia, we recommend appropriate patient selection and caution when using anticoagulant thromboprophylaxis **(Grade 1A)**.
2. For patients receiving deep peripheral nerve blocks, we recommend that the same cautions considered for neuraxial techniques be applied when using anticoagulant thromboprophylaxis **(Grade 1C)**.

General, Vascular, Gynecologic, Urologic, Laparoscopic, Bariatric, Thoracic, and Coronary Artery Bypass Surgery

General Surgery

1. For low-risk general surgery patients who are undergoing minor procedures and have no additional thromboembolic risk factors, we recommend *against* the use of specific thromboprophylaxis other than early and frequent ambulation **(Grade 1A)**.

2. For moderate-risk general surgery patients who are undergoing a major procedure for benign disease, we recommend thromboprophylaxis with LMWH, low-dose unfractionated heparin (LDUH), or fondaparinux **(each Grade 1A)**.

3. For higher-risk general surgery patients who are undergoing a major procedure for cancer, we recommend thromboprophylaxis with LMWH, LDUH three times a day, or fondaparinux **(each Grade 1A)**.

4. For general surgery patients with multiple risk factors for VTE who are thought to be at particularly high risk, we recommend that a pharmacologic method (ie, LMWH, LDUH three times a day, or fondaparinux) be combined with the optimal use of a mechanical method (ie, GCS and/or IPC) **(Grade 1C)**.

5. For general surgery patients with a high risk of bleeding, we recommend the optimal use of mechanical thromboprophylaxis with properly fitted GCS or IPC **(Grade 1A)**. When the high bleeding risk decreases, we recommend that pharmacologic thromboprophylaxis be substituted for, or added to, the mechanical thromboprophylaxis **(Grade 1C)**.

6. For patients undergoing major general surgical procedures, we recommend that thromboprophylaxis continue until discharge from hospital **(Grade 1A)**. For selected high-risk general surgery patients, including some of those who have undergone major cancer surgery or who have previously experienced VTE, we suggest that continuing thromboprophylaxis after hospital discharge with LMWH for up to 28 days be considered **(Grade 2A)**.

Vascular Surgery

1. For patients undergoing vascular surgery who do not have additional thromboembolic risk factors, we suggest that clinicians *not* routinely use specific thromboprophylaxis other than early and frequent ambulation **(Grade 2B)**.

2. For patients undergoing major vascular surgical procedures who have additional thromboembolic risk factors, we recommend thromboprophylaxis with LMWH, LDUH, or fondaparinux **(Grade 1C)**.

Gynecologic Surgery

1. For low-risk gynecologic surgery patients who are undergoing minor procedures and have no additional risk factors, we recommend *against* the use of specific thromboprophylaxis other than early and frequent ambulation **(Grade 1A)**.

2. For gynecology patients undergoing entirely laparoscopic procedures, we recommend *against* routine thromboprophylaxis, other than early and frequent ambulation **(Grade 1B)**.

3. For gynecology patients undergoing entirely laparoscopic procedures in whom additional VTE risk factors are present, we recommend the use of thromboprophylaxis with one or more of LMWH, LDUH, IPC, or GCS **(Grade 1C)**.

4. For all patients undergoing major gynecologic surgery, we recommend that thromboprophylaxis be used routinely **(Grade 1A)**.

5. For patients undergoing major gynecologic surgery for benign disease who have no additional risk factors, we recommend LMWH **(Grade 1A)**, LDUH at 5,000 U **(Grade 1A)**, or IPC started just before surgery and used continuously while the patient is not ambulating **(Grade 1B)**.

6. For patients undergoing extensive surgery for malignancy, and for patients with additional VTE risk factors, we recommend routine thromboprophylaxis with LMWH **(Grade 1A)**, or LDUH at 5,000 U three times daily **(Grade 1A)**, or IPC, started just before surgery and used continuously while the patient is not ambulating (Grade 1A). Alternative considerations include a combination of LDUH or LMWH plus mechanical thromboprophylaxis with GCS or IPC, or fondaparinux (all Grade 1C).

7. For patients undergoing major gynecologic procedures, we recommend that thromboprophylaxis continue until discharge from hospital **(Grade 1A)**. For selected high-risk gynecology patients, including some of those who have undergone major cancer surgery or have previously experienced VTE, we suggest that continuing thromboprophylaxis after hospital discharge with LMWH for up to 28 days be considered **(Grade 2C)**.

Urologic Surgery

1. For patients undergoing transurethral or other low-risk urologic procedures, we recommend *against* the use of specific thromboprophylaxis other than early and frequent ambulation **(Grade 1A)**.

2. For all patients undergoing major, open urologic procedures, we recommend that thromboprophylaxis be used routinely **(Grade 1A)**.

3. For patients undergoing major, open urologic procedures, we recommend routine thromboprophylaxis with LDUH twice or three times daily **(Grade 1B)**, GCS and/or IPC started just before surgery and used continuously while the patient is not ambulating **(Grade 1B)**, LMWH **(Grade 1C)**, fondaparinux **(Grade 1C)**, or the combination of a pharmacologic method (ie, LDUH, LMWH, or fondaparinux) with the optimal use of a mechanical method (ie, GCS and/or IPC) **(Grade 1C)**.

4. For urologic surgery patients who are actively bleeding or who are at very high risk for bleeding, we recommend the optimal use of mechanical thromboprophylaxis with GCS and/or IPC, at least until the bleeding risk decreases **(Grade 1A)**. When the high bleeding risk decreases, we recommend that pharmacologic thromboprophylaxis be substituted for, or added to, the mechanical thromboprophylaxis **(Grade 1C)**.

Laparoscopic Surgery

1. For patients undergoing entirely laparoscopic procedures who do not have additional thromboembolic risk factors, we recommend *against* the routine use of thromboprophylaxis, other than early and frequent ambulation **(Grade 1B)**.

2. For patients undergoing laparoscopic procedures, in whom additional VTE risk factors are present, we recommend the use of thromboprophylaxis with one or more of LMWH, LDUH, fondaparinux, IPC, or GCS **(all Grade 1C)**.

Bariatric Surgery

1. For patients undergoing inpatient bariatric surgery, we recommend routine thromboprophylaxis with LMWH, LDUH three times daily, fondaparinux, or the combination of one of these pharmacologic methods with optimally used IPC **(each Grade 1C)**.

2. For patients undergoing inpatient bariatric surgery, we suggest that higher doses of LMWH or LDUH be used than is usual for non-obese patients **(Grade 2C)**.

Thoracic Surgery

1. For patients undergoing major thoracic surgery, we recommend routine thromboprophylaxis with LMWH, LDUH, or fondaparinux **(each Grade 1C)**.

2. For thoracic surgery patients with a high risk of bleeding, we recommend the optimal use of mechanical thromboprophylaxis with properly fitted GCS and/or IPC **(Grade 1C)**.

Coronary Artery Bypass Surgery

1. For patients undergoing coronary bypass surgery, we recommend the use of thromboprophylaxis with LMWH, LDUH, or optimally used bilateral GCS or IPC **(Grade 1C)**.

2. For patients undergoing coronary bypass surgery, we suggest the use of LMWH over LDUH **(Grade 2B)**.

3. For patients undergoing coronary bypass surgery with a high risk of bleeding, we recommend the optimal use of mechanical thromboprophylaxis with properly fitted bilateral GCS or IPC **(Grade 1C)**.

ORTHOPEDIC SURGERY

Elective Hip Replacement

1. For patients undergoing elective total hip replacement (THR), we recommend the routine use of one of the following anticoagulant options: (1) LMWH (at a usual high-risk dose started 12 hours before surgery or 12 to 24 hours after surgery, or 4 to 6 hours after surgery at half the usual high-risk dose and then increasing to the usual high-risk dose the following day); (2) fondaparinux (2.5 mg started 6 to 24 hours after surgery); or (3) adjusted-dose VKA started preoperatively or the evening of the surgical day (INR target: 2.5; INR range: 2.0 to 3.0) **(all Grade 1A)**.

2. For patients undergoing THR, we recommended *against* the use of any of the following: aspirin, dextran, LDUH, GCS, or VFP as the sole method of thromboprophylaxis **(all Grade 1A)**.

3. For patients undergoing THR who have a high risk of bleeding, we recommend the optimal use of mechanical thromboprophylaxis with the VFP or IPC **(Grade 1A)**. When the high bleeding risk decreases, we recommend that pharmacologic thromboprophylaxis be substituted for, or added to, the mechanical thromboprophylaxis **(Grade 1C)**.

Elective Knee Replacement

1. For patients undergoing TKR, we recommend routine thromboprophylaxis using LMWH (at the usual high-risk dose), fondaparinux, or adjusted-dose VKA (INR target: 2.5; INR range: 2.0 to 3.0) **(all Grade 1A)**.

2. For patients undergoing TKR, the optimal use of IPC is an alternative option to anticoagulant thromboprophylaxis **(Grade 1B)**.

3. For patients undergoing TKR, we recommend *against* the use of any of the following as the only method of thromboprophylaxis: aspirin **(Grade 1A)**, LDUH **(Grade 1A)**, or VFP **(Grade 1B)**.

4. For patients undergoing TKR who have a high risk of bleeding, we recommend the optimal use of mechanical thromboprophylaxis with IPC **(Grade 1A)** or VFP **(Grade 1B)**. When the high bleeding risk decreases, we recommend that pharmacologic thromboprophylaxis be substituted for or added to the mechanical thromboprophylaxis **(Grade 1C)**.

Knee Arthroscopy

1. For patients undergoing knee arthroscopy who do not have additional thromboembolic risk factors, we suggest that clinicians *not* routinely use thromboprophylaxis other than early mobilization **(Grade 2B)**.
2. For patients undergoing arthroscopic knee surgery who have additional thromboembolic risk factors or following a complicated procedure, we recommend thromboprophylaxis with LMWH **(Grade 1B)**.

Hip Fracture Surgery

1. For patients undergoing hip fracture surgery (HFS), we recommend routine thromboprophylaxis using fondaparinux **(Grade 1A)**, LMWH **(Grade 1B)**, adjusted-dose VKA (INR target: 2.5; INR range: 2.0 to 3.0) **(Grade 1B)**, or LDUH **(Grade 1B)**.
2. For patients undergoing HFS, we recommend *against* the use of aspirin alone **(Grade 1A)**.
3. For patients undergoing HFS in whom surgery is likely to be delayed, we recommend that thromboprophylaxis with LMWH or LDUH be initiated during the time between hospital admission and surgery **(Grade 1C)**.
4. For patients undergoing HFS who have a high risk of bleeding, we recommend the optimal use of mechanical thromboprophylaxis **(Grade 1A)**. When the high bleeding risk decreases, we recommend that pharmacologic thromboprophylaxis be substituted for or added to the mechanical thromboprophylaxis **(Grade 1C)**.

OTHER THROMBOPROPHYLAXIS ISSUES IN MAJOR ORTHOPEDIC SURGERY

Commencement of Thromboprophylaxis

1. For patients receiving LMWH as thromboprophylaxis in major orthopedic surgery, we recommend starting either preoperatively or postoperatively **(Grade 1A)**.
2. For patients receiving fondaparinux as thromboprophylaxis in major orthopedic surgery, we recommend starting either 6 to 8 hours after surgery or the next day **(Grade 1A)**.

Screening for DVT before Hospital Discharge

1. For asymptomatic patients following major orthopedic surgery, we recommend *against* the routine use of duplex ultrasound (DUS) screening before hospital discharge **(Grade 1A)**.

Duration of Thromboprophylaxis

1. For patients undergoing THR, TKR, or HFS, we recommend thromboprophylaxis with one of the recommended options for at least 10 days **(Grade 1A)**.
2. For patients undergoing THR, we recommend that thromboprophylaxis be extended beyond 10 days and up to 35 days after surgery **(Grade 1A)**. The recommended options for extended thromboprophylaxis in THR include LMWH **(Grade 1A)**, VKA **(Grade 1B)**, or fondaparinux **(Grade 1C)**.
3. For patients undergoing TKR, we suggest that thromboprophylaxis be extended beyond 10 days and up to 35 days after surgery **(Grade 2B)**. The recommended options for extended thromboprophylaxis in TKR include LMWH **(Grade 1C)**, VKA **(Grade 1C)**, or fondaparinux **(Grade 1C)**.
4. For patients undergoing HFS, we recommend that thromboprophylaxis be extended beyond 10 days and up to 35 days after surgery **(Grade 1A)**. The recommended options for extended thromboprophylaxis in HFS include fondaparinux **(Grade 1A)**, LMWH **(Grade 1C)**, or VKA **(Grade 1C)**.

Elective Spine Surgery

1. For patients undergoing spine surgery who do not have additional thromboembolic risk factors, we suggest that clinicians *not* routinely use specific thromboprophylaxis other than for early and frequent ambulation **(Grade 2C)**.
2. For patients undergoing spine surgery who have additional thromboembolic risk factors, such as advanced age, malignancy, presence of a neurologic deficit, previous VTE, or an anterior surgical approach, we recommend that one of the following thromboprophylaxis options be used: postoperative LDUH **(Grade 1B)**, postoperative LMWH **(Grade 1B)**, or optimal use of perioperative IPC **(Grade 1B)**. An alternative consideration is GCS **(Grade 2B)**.
3. For patients undergoing spine surgery who have multiple risk factors for VTE, we suggest that a pharmacologic method (ie, LDUH or LMWH) be combined with the optimal use of a mechanical method (ie, GCS and/or IPC) **(Grade 2C)**.

Isolated Lower Extremity Injuries Distal to the Knee

1. For patients with isolated lower extremity injuries distal to the knee, we suggest that clinicians do *not* routinely use thromboprophylaxis **(Grade 2A)**.

Neurosurgery

1. For patients undergoing major neurosurgery, we recommend that thromboprophylaxis be used routinely **(Grade 1A)**, with optimal use of IPC **(Grade 1A)**. Acceptable alternatives to IPC are postoperative LMWH **(Grade 2A)** or LDUH **(Grade 2B)**.
2. For patients undergoing major neurosurgery who have a particularly high thrombosis risk, we suggest that a mechanical method (ie, GCS and/or IPC) be combined with a pharmacologic method (ie, postoperative LMWH or LDUH) **(Grade 2B)**.

Trauma, Spinal Cord Injury, Burns

Trauma

1. For all major trauma patients, we recommend routine thromboprophylaxis, if possible **(Grade 1A)**.
2. For major trauma patients, in the absence of a major contraindication, we recommend that clinicians use LMWH thromboprophylaxis starting as soon as it is considered safe to do so **(Grade 1A)**. An acceptable alternative is the combination of LMWH and the optimal use of a mechanical method of thromboprophylaxis **(Grade 1B)**.
3. For major trauma patients, if LMWH thromboprophylaxis is contraindicated due to active bleeding or high risk for clinically important bleeding, we recommend that mechanical thromboprophylaxis with IPC, or possibly with GCS alone, be used **(Grade 1B)**. When the high bleeding risk decreases, we recommend that pharmacologic thromboprophylaxis be substituted for or added to the mechanical thromboprophylaxis **(Grade 1C)**.
4. In trauma patients, we recommend *against* routine DUS screening for asymptomatic DVT **(Grade 1B)**. We do recommend DUS screening in patients who are at high risk for VTE (eg, in the presence of a spinal cord injury [SCI], lower extremity or pelvic fracture, or major head injury) and who have received suboptimal thromboprophylaxis or no thromboprophylaxis **(Grade 1C)**.
5. For trauma patients, we recommend *against* the use of an inferior vena-caval (IVC) filter as thromboprophylaxis **(Grade 1C)**.
6. For major trauma patients, we recommend the continuation of thromboprophylaxis until hospital discharge, including the period of inpa-

tient rehabilitation **(Grade 1C)**. For trauma patients with impaired mobility who undergo inpatient rehabilitation, we suggest continuing thromboprophylaxis with LMWH or VKA (target INR: 2.5; range: 2.0 to 3.0) **(Grade 2C)**.

Acute Spinal Cord Injury

1. For all patients with acute SCI, we recommend that routine thromboprophylaxis be provided **(Grade 1A)**.
2. For patients with acute SCI, we recommend thromboprophylaxis with LMWH, commenced once primary hemostasis is evident **(Grade 1B)**. Alternatives include the combined use of IPC and either LDUH **(Grade 1B)** or LWMH **(Grade 1C)**.
3. For patients with acute SCI, we recommend the optimal use of IPC and/or GCS if anticoagulant thromboprophylaxis is contraindicated because of high bleeding risk early after injury **(Grade 1A)**. When the high bleeding risk decreases, we recommend that pharmacologic thromboprophylaxis be substituted for or added to the mechanical thromboprophylaxis **(Grade 1C)**.
4. For patients with an incomplete SCI associated with evidence of a spinal hematoma on computed tomography (CT) or magnetic resonance imaging (MRI), we recommend the use of mechanical thromboprophylaxis instead of anticoagulant thromboprophylaxis, at least for the first few days after injury **(Grade 1C)**.
5. Following acute SCI, we recommend *against* the use of LDUH alone **(Grade 1A)**.
6. For patients with SCI, we recommend *against* the use of an IVC filter as thromboprophylaxis **(Grade 1C)**.
7. For patients undergoing rehabilitation following acute SCI, we recommend the continuation of LMWH thromboprophylaxis or conversion to an oral VKA (target INR: 2.5; range: 2.0 to 3.0) **(Grade 1C)**.

Burns

1. For burn patients who have additional risk factors for VTE, including one or more of the following: advanced age, morbid obesity, extensive or lower extremity burns, concomitant lower extremity trauma, use of a femoral venous catheter, and/or prolonged immobility, we recommend routine thromboprophylaxis, if possible **(Grade 1A)**.
2. For burn patients who have additional risk factors for VTE, if there are no contraindications, we recommend the use of either LMWH or LDUH, starting as soon as it is considered safe to do so **(Grade 1C)**.

3. For burn patients who have a high bleeding risk, we recommend mechanical thromboprophylaxis with GCS and/or IPC until the bleeding risk decreases **(Grade 1A)**.

Medical Conditions

1. For acutely ill medical patients admitted to hospital with congestive heart failure or severe respiratory disease, or who are confined to bed and have one or more additional risk factors, including active cancer, previous VTE, sepsis, acute neurologic disease, or inflammatory bowel disease, we recommend thromboprophylaxis with LMWH **(Grade 1A)**, LDUH **(Grade 1A)**, or fondaparinux **(Grade 1A)**.
2. For medical patients with risk factors for VTE, and in whom there is a contraindication to anticoagulant thromboprophylaxis, we recommend the optimal use of mechanical thromboprophylaxis with GCS or IPC **(Grade 1A)**.

Cancer Patients

1. For cancer patients undergoing surgical procedures, we recommend routine thromboprophylaxis that is appropriate for the type of surgery **(Grade 1A)**. Refer to the recommendations in the relevant surgical subsections.
2. For cancer patients who are bedridden with an acute medical illness, we recommend routine thromboprophylaxis as advised for other high-risk medical patients **(Grade 1A)**.
3. For cancer patients with indwelling central venous catheters, we recommend that clinicians *not* use either prophylactic doses of LMWH **(Grade 1B)** or mini-dose warfarin **(Grade 1B)** to try to prevent catheter-related thrombosis.
4. For cancer patients receiving chemotherapy or hormonal therapy, we recommend *against* the routine use of thromboprophylaxis for the primary prevention of VTE **(Grade 1C)**.
5. For cancer patients, we recommend *against* the routine use of primary thromboprophylaxis to try to improve survival **(Grade 1B)**.

Critical Care

1. For patients admitted to a critical care unit, we recommend routine assessment for VTE risk and routine thromboprophylaxis for most **(Grade 1A).**
2. For critical care patients who are at moderate risk for VTE (eg, medically ill or postoperative general surgery patients), we recommend using LMWH or LDUH thromboprophylaxis **(Grade 1A)**.

3. For critical care patients who are at higher risk (eg, following major trauma or orthopedic surgery), we recommend LMWH thromboprophylaxis **(Grade 1A)**.
4. For critical care patients who are at high risk for bleeding, we recommend the optimal use of mechanical thromboprophylaxis with GCS and/or IPC, at least until the bleeding risk decreases **(Grade 1A)**. When the high bleeding risk decreases, we recommend that pharmacologic thromboprophylaxis be substituted for or added to the mechanical thromboprophylaxis **(Grade 1C)**.

Long-Distance Travel
1. For travelers who are taking flights longer than 8 hours, we recommend the following general measures: avoidance of constrictive clothing around the lower extremities or waist, maintenance of adequate hydration, and frequent calf muscle contraction **(Grade 1C)**.
2. For long-distance travelers with additional risk factors for VTE, we recommend the general measures listed above. If active thromboprophylaxis is considered because of a perceived high risk of VTE, we suggest the use of properly fitted, below-knee GCS, providing 15 to 30 mm Hg of pressure at the ankle **(Grade 2C)**, or a single prophylactic dose of LMWH, injected prior to departure **(Grade 2C)**.
3. For long-distance travelers, we recommend *against* the use of aspirin for VTE prevention **(Grade 1B)**.

10 ANTITHROMBOTIC THERAPY FOR VENOUS THROMBOEMBOLIC DISEASE

Patients with venous thromboembolic disease have a high risk of recurrence if untreated or if treated with subtherapeutic doses of anticoagulants. Recurrent pulmonary embolism can be fatal, or death can occur from massive pulmonary embolism. The objectives of therapy are to prevent thrombus extension, early and late recurrences of venous thrombosis and pulmonary embolism (including fatal PE) and to prevent the post-thrombotic syndrome. The risk of recurrence (including fatal recurrence) is reduced markedly if anticoagulants are started promptly and in appropriate dosages. The risk of developing post-thrombotic syndrome can be reduced by the early application of compression stockings. Selected patients with thromboembolic pulmonary hypertension respond to pulmonary thromboendarterectomy.

INITIAL TREATMENT

Anticoagulant therapy is the mainstay of treatment for DVT. It prevents thrombus extension and early and late recurrences of VTE. Patients with DVT should be treated with anticoagulants as soon as the diagnosis is confirmed, or if the clinical suspicion is high, it should be started without delay. The following options are available for the initial treatment of DVT: (1) low-molecular-weight heparin (LMWH), given subcutaneously without monitoring; (2) intravenous (IV) unfractionated heparin (UFH) given with monitoring; (3) subcutaneous (SC) UFH given with monitoring; (4) weight-based SC UFH given without monitoring; and (5) fondaparinux, given subcutaneously without monitoring.

Warfarin is started at the same time, and the parenteral agent is discontinued after 5 days, provided the INR is 2.0 or above for at least 24 hours. Warfarin is generally started at a dose of 2.5 to 10 mg. Doses of warfarin in the lower range are required in older patients and those with impaired nutrition and with vitamin K deficiency.

If UFH is given intravenously by continuous infusion, the dose is adjusted in response to coagulation monitoring. The starting dose of IV UFH for the treatment of DVT is either (1) a bolus dose of 5,000 U followed by a continuous infusion of at least 30,000 U for the first 24 hours, or (2) a weight adjusted regimen of an 80 U/kg bolus, followed by 18 U/kg/h. With both of these regimens, the dose is adjusted using a standard nomogram to rapidly reach and maintain the activated partial thromboplastin time (APTT) at levels that correspond to therapeutic heparin levels. It is not necessary to increase the UFH infusion dose above 1,667 U/h (corresponding to 40,000 U/d) if the anti-factor Xa heparin level is at least 0.35 U/mL, even if the APTT ratio is below the therapeutic range.

COMPARISONS OF DIFFERENT PARENTERAL ANTICOAGULANTS

Low-Molecular-Weight Heparin

Weight-adjusted doses of LMWH can be given subcutaneously once or twice daily without laboratory monitoring in the majority of patients. However, in severe renal failure or pregnancy, LMWH dose adjustment may be required using anti-factor Xa heparin levels. A target range (4 hours after injection) of 0.6 to 1.0 IU/mL is suggested for twice-daily administration, and a target range of 1.0 to 2.0 IU/mL is suggested for once-daily administration.

Results of a meta-analysis indicate that, compared to IV UFH given with monitoring, weight-adjusted LMWH given SC is associated with significantly fewer thrombotic complications (3.6% vs 5.4%), significantly less major bleeding (1.2% vs 2.0%) and fewer deaths (4.5% vs 6.0%). The mortality advantage with LMWH appeared to be confined to patients with cancer.

LMWH preparations appear to show similar efficacy and safety with once- and twice-daily administration, with outpatients and inpatients administration, and with the use of different preparations.

Subcutaneous Unfractionated Heparin

SC UFH given twice daily appears to be as safe and effective as continuous IV infusion. Two SC regimens have been shown to be effective and safe: (1) an initial IV bolus of about 5,000 U followed by an SC dose of about 17,500 U twice a day on the first day, with subsequent adjustment based on the APTT or on anti-factor Xa activity, and (2) fixed-dose, unmonitored SC UFH in a dose of 333 U/kg followed by a twice-daily dose of 250 U/kg.

Fondaparinux

Once-daily fondaparinux given subcutaneously (7.5 mg if patient's weight is 50 to 100 kg; 5 mg if patient's weight is less than 50 kg; 10 mg if patient's weight is greater than 100 kg) is as effective and safe as twice-daily SC LMWH (enoxaparin 1 mg/kg).

THROMBUS REMOVAL FOR ACUTE DVT

There is emerging evidence that active removal of the thrombus in patients with acute DVT might improve patient outcomes in selected patients with iliofemoral DVT. To date, however, experience with these techniques is limited. Newer techniques include (1) catheter-directed thrombolysis (CDT) used either alone or with intravascular stenting or with mechanical thrombus fragmentation, and (2) mechanical thrombus fragmentation used alone, with or without aspiration. Older approaches include systemic thrombolytic therapy and thrombectomy.

Systemic Thrombolytic Therapy

There are limited data comparing systemic thrombolytic therapy with anticoagulant therapy alone in acute DVT. Systemic thrombolytic therapy achieved a higher frequency of complete or significant lysis (as assessed by early repeat phlebography) and appeared to reduce post-thrombotic morbidity (relative risk: 0.7; 95% CI: 0.5 to 0.9), but at the cost of increased early significant or major bleeding (relative risk: 1.7; 95% CI: 1.04 to 2.9).

Operative Venous Thrombectomy

Although data on operative thrombectomy are limited, this approach might reduce acute symptoms and post-thrombotic morbidity in selected patients with acute iliofemoral DVT. After thrombectomy, patients should be treated with anticoagulant therapy in the same manner as those who do not undergo venous thrombectomy.

Caval Filters

Inferior vena caval filter insertion has been evaluated in patients who were also anticoagulated. In these patients, the deployment of a permanent filter reduced the short- and long-term risk of PE but at the cost of an increase in the risk of DVT at 2 years.

When used without anticoagulant therapy, venous thrombosis at the site of filter insertion sites occurs in about 10% of patients. If anticoagulant therapy is temporarily contraindicated because of bleeding, a retrievable filter can be inserted and removed when it is safe to start anticoagulant therapy. However, the risks and benefits of using a retrievable filter compared with a permanent filter in this setting are uncertain. Based on current data, the use of vena cava filters should be limited to patients with acute proximal DVT if anticoagulant therapy is not possible because of the risk of bleeding. These patients should receive a conventional course of anticoagulant therapy if their risk of bleeding resolves.

LONG-TERM TREATMENT OF ACUTE DEEP VEIN THROMBOSIS

Anticoagulant therapy is continued for a minimum of 3 months and longer in patients with a high risk of recurrence.

The risk of recurrent VTE after stopping vitamin K antagonist (VKA) therapy is much lower if the index event was provoked by a reversible risk factor than if the episode was unprovoked (also called idiopathic VTE). The risk of recurrence when stopping anticoagulant therapy is also lower if the DVT is confined to the distal veins. Reversible provoking risk factors include: major factors, such as surgery, hospitalization, or plaster cast immobilization, all within 1 month; and minor factors, such as estrogen therapy, pregnancy, prolonged travel (eg, longer than 8 hours). The risk of recurrent thrombosis is also lower after a first episode of VTE rather than a second or subsequent episode of VTE.

Based on these considerations, 3 months of anticoagulant therapy are sufficient for patients with DVT secondary to a transient (reversible) risk factor or in those who have had a single episode of isolated distal DVT that is unprovoked. Patients with unprovoked proximal DVT should be treated with anticoagulants for at least 3 months, at which time they should be evaluated for the risk to benefit of long-term therapy. Long-term treatment is indicated if there are no risk factors for bleeding and good anticoagulant monitoring is achievable.

Patients who have had a second episode of unprovoked VTE should receive long-term treatment.

LMWH is more effective than VKA in patients with DVT and cancer. In such patients, LMWH is given for the first 3 to 6 months of long-term anticoagulant therapy and is followed by either VKA or LMWH indefinitely or until the cancer is resolved.

For most patients, the optimal intensity of anticoagulant therapy is an INR of 2.5 (range 2.0 to 3.0). However, the intensity can be lowered to an INR range of 1.5 to 1.9 in patients with unprovoked VTE who have a strong preference for less frequent INR testing.

PREVENTION OF POST-THROMBOTIC SYNDROME

Post-thrombotic syndrome (PTS) occurs in 20 to 50% of patients after acute DVT. There is evidence that the incidence and severity of PTS is reduced by the use of elastic compression stockings that are applied soon after the acute episode of DVT.

Patients with severe PTS might derive benefit from treatment with intermittent pneumatic compression at a pressure of 40 mm Hg. There is also evidence that patients with venous ulcers might benefit from pharmacotherapy with pentoxifylline, flavonoids, or sulodexide.

INITIAL TREATMENT OF PULMONARY EMBOLISM

The treatment of DVT and PE is similar, with most PE patients receiving anticoagulant therapy. The risk of early death is much greater in patients presenting with PE than after DVT, and if recurrences occur in VTE patients, they are three times more likely to be PE after an initial PE than after an initial DVT. For these reasons, more aggressive initial and long-term therapy is more often indicated in patients with PE than in those with DVT.

Thrombolytic therapy with t-PA is indicated for the treatment of PE associated with hemodynamic compromise, but there is less certainty about the role of thrombolytic therapy in patients with normal systemic arterial pressure.

Treatment of massive PE with interventional catheterization techniques or traditional pulmonary embolectomy can prove life saving in desperate situations. Pulmonary thromboendarterectomy can reduce the severity of, and sometimes cure, chronic thromboembolic pulmonary hypertension (CTPH), a condition that occurs more frequently after acute PE than was previously believed.

SUPERFICIAL THROMBOPHLEBITIS

A number of small studies have reported that the following approaches are effective for the treatment of peripheral vein infusion thrombophlebitis: diclofenac emulsion gel, oral diclofenac, heparin sodium gel, and Essaven gel.

In patients with spontaneous superficial vein thrombosis, prophylactic or intermediate doses of LMWH or intermediate doses of UFH for at least 4 weeks have been shown to be effective.

UPPER EXTREMITY DVT

Both the short-term and long-term treatment of patients with acute upper extremity DVT (UEDVT) is similar to that of lower extremity DVT. We recommend initial treatment with therapeutic doses of LMWH, UFH, or fondaparinux as described for leg DVT.

RECOMMENDATIONS

Initial Anticoagulation of Acute DVT of the Leg

1. For patients with objectively confirmed DVT, we recommend acute treatment with SC LMWH **(Grade 1A)**, IV UFH **(Grade 1A)**, monitored SC UFH **(Grade 1A)**, fixed-dose SC UFH **(Grade 1A)**, or SC fondaparinux **(Grade 1A)** rather than no such acute treatment.
2. For patients with a high clinical suspicion of DVT, we recommend treatment with anticoagulants while awaiting the outcome of diagnostic tests **(Grade 1C)**.
3. In patients with acute DVT, we recommend initial treatment with LMWH, UFH, or fondaparinux for at least 5 days and until the INR is 2.0 or greater for 24 hours **(Grade 1C)**.
4. In patients with acute DVT, we recommend initiation of VKA together with LMWH, UFH, or fondaparinux on the first treatment day rather than delayed initiation of VKA **(Grade 1A)**.

IV UFH for the Initial Treatment of DVT

1. In patients with acute DVT, if IV UFH is chosen, we recommend that, after an initial IV bolus (80 U/kg or 5,000 U) it is administered by continuous infusion (initially at a dose of 18 U/kg/h or 1,300 U/h) with dose adjustment to achieve and maintain an APTT prolongation that corresponds to plasma heparin levels of 0.3 to 0.7 IU/mL anti-factor Xa activity by the amidolytic assay, rather than administration as IV boluses throughout treatment, or administration without coagulation monitoring **(Grade 1C)**.

SC UFH Compared With IV Heparin for the Initial Treatment of DVT

1. In patients with acute DVT, if monitored SC UFH is chosen, we recommend an initial dose of 17,500 U, or a weight-adjusted dose of about 250 U/kg, twice daily, with dose adjustment to achieve and maintain an APTT prolongation that corresponds to plasma heparin levels of 0.3 to 0.7 IU/mL anti-factor Xa activity when measured 6 hours after injection, rather than starting with a smaller initial dose **(Grade 1C)**.

2. In patients with acute DVT, if fixed-dose unmonitored SC UFH is chosen, we recommend an initial dose of 333 U/kg followed by a twice-daily dose of 250 U/kg rather than non–weight-based dosing **(Grade 1C)**.

LMWH for the Initial Treatment of DVT

1. In patients with acute DVT, we recommend initial treatment with LMWH SC once or twice a day, as an outpatient, if possible **(Grade 1C),** or as an inpatient, if necessary **(Grade 1A)**, rather than treatment with IV UFH.

2. In patients with acute DVT treated with LMWH, we recommend against routine monitoring with anti-factor Xa level measurements **(Grade 1A)**.

3. In patients with acute DVT and severe renal failure, we suggest UFH over LMWH **(Grade 2C)**.

Catheter-Directed Thrombolysis for Acute DVT

1. In selected patients with extensive acute proximal DVT (eg, iliofemoral DVT, symptoms for < 14 days, good functional status, life expectancy of ≥ 1 year) who have a low risk of bleeding, we suggest that catheter-directed thrombolysis may be used to reduce acute symptoms and post-thrombotic morbidity if appropriate expertise and resources are available **(Grade 2B)**.

2. After successful catheter-directed thrombolysis in patients with acute DVT, we suggest correction of underlying venous lesions using balloon angioplasty and stents **(Grade 2C)**.

3. We suggest pharmacomechanical thrombolysis (eg, with inclusion of thrombus fragmentation and/or aspiration) in preference to catheter-directed thrombolysis alone to shorten treatment time if appropriate expertise and resources are available **(Grade 2C)**.

4. After successful catheter-directed thrombolysis in patients with acute DVT, we recommend the same intensity and duration of anticoagulant therapy as for comparable patients who do not undergo catheter-directed thrombolysis **(Grade 1C)**.

Systemic Thrombolytic Therapy for Acute DVT

1. In selected patients with extensive proximal DVT (eg, symptoms for < 14 days, good functional status, life expectancy of ≥ 1 year) who have a low risk of bleeding, we suggest that systemic thrombolytic therapy may be used to reduce acute symptoms and post-thrombotic morbidity if catheter-directed thrombolysis is not available **(Grade 2C)**.

Percutaneous Venous Thrombectomy

1. In patients with acute DVT, we suggest they should *not* be treated with percutaneous mechanical thrombectomy alone **(Grade 2C)**.

Operative Venous Thrombectomy for Acute DVT

1. In selected patients with acute iliofemoral DVT (eg, symptoms for < 7 days, good functional status, and life expectancy of ≥ 1 year), we suggest that operative venous thrombectomy may be used to reduce acute symptoms and post-thrombotic morbidity if appropriate expertise and resources are available **(Grade 2B)**. If such patients do not have a high risk of bleeding, we suggest that catheter-directed thrombolysis is usually preferable to operative venous thrombectomy **(Grade 2C)**.

2. In patients who undergo operative venous thrombectomy, we recommend the same intensity and duration of anticoagulant therapy afterwards as for comparable patients who do not undergo venous thrombectomy **(Grade 1C)**.

Vena Caval Filters for the Initial Treatment of DVT

1. For patients with DVT, we recommend against the routine use of a vena caval filter in addition to anticoagulants **(Grade 1A)**.

2. For patients with acute proximal DVT, if anticoagulant therapy is not possible because of the risk of bleeding, we recommend placement of an inferior vena caval filter **(Grade 1C)**.

3. For patients with acute DVT who have an inferior vena caval filter inserted as an alternative to anticoagulation, we recommend that they should subsequently receive a conventional course of anticoagulant therapy if their risk of bleeding resolves **(Grade 1C)**.

Immobilization for the Treatment of Acute DVT

1. In patients with acute DVT, we recommend early ambulation in preference to initial bed rest when this is feasible **(Grade 1A)**.

Duration of Anticoagulant Therapy

1. For patients with DVT secondary to a transient (reversible) risk factor, we recommend treatment with VKA for 3 months over treatment for shorter periods **(Grade 1A)**.

2. For patients with unprovoked DVT, we recommend treatment with VKA for at least 3 months **(Grade 1A)**. We recommend that, after 3 months of anticoagulant therapy, all patients with unprovoked DVT should be evaluated for the risk-benefit ratio of long-term therapy **(Grade 1C)**. For patients with a first unprovoked DVT that is a proximal DVT and in whom risk factors for bleeding are absent and for whom good anticoagulant monitoring is achievable, we recommend long-term treatment **(Grade 1A)**.

3. For patients with a second episode of unprovoked DVT, we recommend long-term treatment **(Grade 1A)**. For patients with a first isolated distal DVT that is unprovoked, we suggest that 3 months of anticoagulant therapy is sufficient, rather than indefinite therapy **(Grade 2B)**.

4. For patients with DVT and cancer, we recommend LMWH for the first 3 to 6 months of long-term anticoagulant therapy **(Grade 1A)**. For these patients, we recommend subsequent anticoagulant therapy with VKA or LMWH indefinitely or until the cancer is resolved **(Grade 1C)**.

5. In patients who receive long-term anticoagulant treatment, the risk-benefit ratio of continuing such treatment should be reassessed in the individual patient at periodic intervals **(Grade 1C)**.

Intensity of Anticoagulant Effect

1. In patients with DVT, we recommend that the dosage of VKA be adjusted to maintain a target INR of 2.5 (INR range: 2.0 to 3.0) for all treatment durations **(Grade 1A)**. For patients with unprovoked DVT who have a strong preference for less frequent INR testing to monitor their therapy, after the first 3 months of conventional-intensity anticoagulation (INR range: 2.0 to 3.0), we recommend low-intensity therapy (INR range: 1.5 to 1.9) with less frequent INR monitoring over stopping treatment **(Grade 1A)**. We recommend against high intensity VKA therapy (INR range: 3.1 to 4.0) compared to an INR range of 2.0 to 3.0 **(Grade 1A)**.

Treatment of Asymptomatic DVT of the Leg

1. In patients who are unexpectedly found to have asymptomatic DVT, we recommend the same initial and long-term anticoagulation as for comparable patients with symptomatic DVT **(Grade 1C)**.

Elastic Stockings and Compression Bandages to Prevent PTS

1. For a patient who has had a symptomatic proximal DVT, we recommend the use of an elastic compression stocking with an ankle pressure

gradient of 30 to 40 mm Hg, if feasible **(Grade 1A)**. Compression therapy, which may include use of bandages acutely, should be started as soon as feasible after starting anticoagulant therapy and should be continued for a minimum of 2 years, and longer if patients have symptoms of the post-thrombotic syndrome. (Note: Feasibility, both acutely and long-term, refers to the ability of patients and their caregivers to apply and remove stockings.)

Physical Treatment of PTS Without Venous Leg Ulcers

1. For patients with severe edema of the leg due to PTS, we suggest a course of intermittent pneumatic compression **(Grade 2B)**.
2. For patients with mild edema of the leg due to PTS, we suggest the use of elastic compression stockings **(Grade 2C)**.

Physical Treatment of Venous Leg Ulcers

1. In patients with venous ulcers resistant to healing with wound care and compression, we suggest the addition of intermittent pneumatic compression (IPC) **(Grade 2B)**.

Hyperbaric Oxygen and the Management of Patients With Venous Ulcers

1. For patients with venous ulcers, we suggest that hyperbaric oxygen *not* be used **(Grade 2B)**.

Pentoxifylline

1. In patients with venous leg ulcers, we suggest pentoxifylline 400 mg orally three times a day in addition to local care and compression and/or IPC **(Grade 2B)**.

Micronized Purified Flavonoid Fraction or Sulodexide for the Treatment of Venous Leg Ulcers

1. In patients with persistent venous ulcers, we suggest that rutosides, in the form of micronized purified flavonoid fraction given orally, or sulodexide given intramuscularly and then orally, be added to local care and compression **(Grade 2B)**.

IV or SC UFH, SC LMWH, SC Fondaparinux, and VKA for the Initial Treatment of PE

1. For patients with objectively confirmed PE, we recommend acute treatment with SC LMWH **(Grade 1A)**, IV UFH **(Grade 1A)**, monitored SC UFH **(Grade 1A)**, fixed-dose SC UFH **(Grade 1A)**, or SC fondaparinux **(Grade 1A)** rather than no such acute treatment.

Patients with acute PE should also be routinely assessed for treatment with thrombolytic therapy

2. For patients in whom there is a high clinical suspicion of PE, we recommend treatment with anticoagulants while awaiting the outcome of diagnostic tests **(Grade 1C)**.

3. In patients with acute PE, we recommend initial treatment with LMWH, UFH, or fondaparinux for at least 5 days and until the INR is 2.0 or greater for at least 24 hours **(Grade 1C)**.

4. In patients with acute PE, we recommend initiation of VKA together with LMWH, UFH, or fondaparinux on the first treatment day rather than delayed initiation of VKA **(Grade 1A)**.

5. In patients with acute PE, if IV UFH is chosen, we recommend that, after an initial IV bolus (80 U/kg or 5,000 U), it be administered by continuous infusion (initially at dose of 18 U/kg/h or 1,300 U/h) with dose adjustment to achieve and maintain an APTT prolongation that corresponds to plasma heparin levels of 0.3 to 0.7 IU/mL anti-factor Xa activity by the amidolytic assay, rather than administration as IV boluses throughout treatment, or administration without coagulation monitoring **(Grade 1C)**.

6. In patients with acute PE, if monitored SC UFH is chosen, we recommend an initial dose of 17,500 U, or a weight-adjusted dose of about 250 U/kg, twice daily, with dose adjustment to achieve and maintain an APTT prolongation that corresponds to plasma heparin levels of 0.3 to 0.7 IU/mL anti-factor Xa activity when measured 6 hours after injection, rather than starting with a smaller initial dose **(Grade 1C)**.

7. In patients with acute PE, if fixed-dose, unmonitored SC UFH is chosen, we recommend an initial dose of 333 U/kg followed by a twice-daily dose of 250 U/kg rather than non–weight-based dosing **(Grade 1C)**.

8. In patients with acute non-massive PE, we recommend initial treatment with LMWH over IV UFH **(Grade 1A)**. In patients with massive PE, in other situations where there is concern about SC absorption, or in patients in whom thrombolytic therapy is being considered or planned, we recommend IV UFH over SC LMWH, SC fondaparinux, or SC UFH **(Grade 2C)**.

9. In patients with acute PE treated with LMWH, we recommend against routine monitoring with anti-factor Xa level measurements **(Grade 1A)**.

10. In patients with acute PE and severe renal failure, we suggest UFH over LMWH **(Grade 2C)**.

Systemically and Locally Administered Thrombolytic Therapy for PE

1. All PE patients should undergo rapid risk stratification **(Grade 1C)**. For patients with evidence of hemodynamic compromise, we recommend use of thrombolytic therapy unless there are major contraindications due to bleeding risk **(Grade 1B)**. Thrombolysis in these patients should not be delayed, because irreversible cardiogenic shock may ensue. In selected high-risk patients without hypotension who are judged to have a low risk of bleeding, we suggest administration of thrombolytic therapy **(Grade 2B)**. The decision to use thrombolytic therapy depends on the clinician's assessment of PE severity, prognosis, and risk of bleeding. For the majority of patients with PE, we recommend against using thrombolytic therapy **(Grade 1B)**.

2. In patients with acute PE, when a thrombolytic agent is used, we recommend that treatment be administered via a peripheral vein rather than placing a pulmonary artery catheter to administer treatment **(Grade 1B)**.

3. In patients with acute PE, with administration of thrombolytic therapy, we recommend use of regimens with short infusion times (eg, a 2-hour infusion) over those with prolonged infusion times (eg, a 24-hour infusion) **(Grade 1B)**.

Catheter Extraction or Fragmentation for the Initial Treatment of PE

1. For most patients with PE, we recommend against use of interventional catheterization techniques **(Grade 1C)**. In selected highly compromised patients who are unable to receive thrombolytic therapy because of bleeding risk, or whose critical status does not allow sufficient time for systemic thrombolytic therapy to be effective, we suggest use of interventional catheterization techniques if appropriate expertise is available **(Grade 2C)**.

Pulmonary Embolectomy for the Initial Treatment of PE

1. In selected highly compromised patients who are unable to receive thrombolytic therapy because of bleeding risk, or whose critical status does not allow sufficient time for systemic thrombolytic therapy to be effective, we suggest that pulmonary embolectomy may be used if appropriate expertise is available **(Grade 2C)**.

Vena Caval Filters for the Initial Treatment of PE

1. For most patients with PE, we recommend against the routine use of a vena caval filter in addition to anticoagulants **(Grade 1A)**.

2. In patients with acute PE, if anticoagulant therapy is not possible because of risk of bleeding, we recommend placement of an inferior vena caval filter **(Grade 1C)**.
3. For patients with acute PE who have an inferior vena caval filter inserted as an alternative to anticoagulation, we recommend that they should subsequently receive a conventional course of anticoagulant therapy if their risk of bleeding resolves **(Grade 1C)**.

Long-term Treatment of Acute Pulmonary Embolism

1. For patients with PE secondary to a transient (reversible) risk factor, we recommend treatment with VKA for 3 months over treatment for shorter periods **(Grade 1A)**.
2. For patients with unprovoked PE, we recommend treatment with VKA for at least 3 months **(Grade 1A)**. We recommend that, after 3 months of anticoagulant therapy, all patients with unprovoked PE should be evaluated for the risk-benefit ratio of long-term therapy **(Grade 1C)**. For patients with a first unprovoked episode of PE, and in whom risk factors for bleeding are absent and for whom good anticoagulant monitoring is achievable, we recommend long-term treatment **(Grade 1A)**.
3. For patients with a second episode of unprovoked PE, we recommend long-term treatment **(Grade 1A)**.
4. For patients with PE and cancer, we recommend LMWH for the first 3 to 6 months of long-term anticoagulant therapy **(Grade 1A)**. For these patients, we recommend subsequent anticoagulant therapy with VKA or LMWH long term or until the cancer is resolved **(Grade 1C)**.
5. In patients who receive long-term anticoagulant treatment, the risk-benefit ratio of continuing such treatment should be reassessed in the individual patient at periodic intervals **(Grade 1C)**.
6. In patients with PE, we recommend that the dosage of VKA be adjusted to maintain a target INR of 2.5 (INR range: 2.0 to 3.0) for all treatment durations **(Grade 1A)**. For patients with unprovoked PE who have a strong preference for less frequent INR testing to monitor their therapy, after the first 3 months of conventional-intensity anticoagulation (INR range: 2.0 to 3.0), we recommend low-intensity therapy (INR range: 1.5 to 1.9) with less frequent INR monitoring over stopping treatment **(Grade 1A)**. We recommend against high intensity VKA therapy (INR range: 3.1 to 4.0) compared with an INR range of 2.0 to 3.0 **(Grade 1A)**.
7. In patients who are unexpectedly found to have asymptomatic PE, we recommend the same initial and long-term anticoagulation as for comparable patients with symptomatic PE **(Grade 1C)**.

Pulmonary Thromboendarterectomy, VKA, and Vena Caval Filter for the Treatment of CTPH

1. In selected patients with CTPH, such as those with central disease under the care of an experienced surgical/medical team, we recommend pulmonary thromboendarterectomy **(Grade 1C)**.
2. For all patients with CTPH, we recommend life-long treatment with VKA targeted to an INR of 2.0 to 3.0 **(Grade 1C)**.
3. For patients with CTPH undergoing pulmonary thromboendarterectomy, we suggest the placement of a permanent vena caval filter before, or at the time of, the procedure **(Grade 2C)**.
4. For patients with inoperable CTPH, we suggest referral to a center with expertise in pulmonary hypertension so that patients can be evaluated for alternative treatments, such as vasodilator therapy or balloon pulmonary angioplasty **(Grade 2C)**.

Treatment of Infusion Thrombophlebitis

1. For patients with symptomatic infusion thrombophlebitis as a complication of IV infusion, we suggest oral diclofenac or another non-steroidal anti-inflammatory drug (NSAID) **(Grade 2B)**, topical diclofenac gel **(Grade 2B)**, or heparin gel **(Grade 2B)** until resolution of symptoms or for up to 2 weeks. We recommend against the use of systemic anticoagulation **(Grade 1C)**.

Treatment of Superficial Vein Thrombosis

1. For patients with spontaneous superficial vein thrombosis, we suggest prophylactic or intermediate doses of LMWH **(Grade 2B)** or intermediate doses of UFH **(Grade 2B)** for at least 4 weeks. We suggest that, as an alternative to 4 weeks of LMWH or UFH, VKA (target INR: 2.5; range: 2.0 to 3.0) can be overlapped with 5 days of UFH and LMWH and continued for 4 weeks **(Grade 2C)**. We suggest that oral NSAIDs should not be used in addition to anticoagulation **(Grade 2B)**. We recommend medical treatment with anticoagulants over surgical treatment **(Grade 1B)**.

Remark: It is likely that less extensive superficial vein thrombosis (ie, where the affected venous segment is short in length or further from the saphenofemoral junction) does not require treatment with anticoagulants. It is reasonable to use oral or topical NSAIDs for symptom control in such cases.

IV UFH or LMWH for the Initial Treatment of Upper Limb Deep Venous Thrombosis

1. For patients with acute UEDVT, we recommend initial treatment with therapeutic doses of LMWH, UFH, or fondaparinux as described for leg DVT (see section 1 below) **(Grade 1C)**.

Thrombolytic Therapy for the Initial Treatment of UEDVT

1. For most patients with acute UEDVT, we recommend against the routine use of systemic or catheter-directed thrombolytic therapy **(Grade 1C)**.
2. In selected patients with acute UEDVT (eg, in those with a low risk of bleeding and severe symptoms of recent onset), we suggest a short course of catheter-directed thrombolytic therapy for initial treatment, if appropriate expertise and resources are available **(Grade 2C)**.

Catheter Extraction, Surgical Thrombectomy, Transluminal Angioplasty, Stent Placement, Staged Approach of Lysis Followed by Interventional or Surgical Procedure, Superior Vena Caval Filter Insertion for the Initial Treatment of UEDVT

1. For most patients with acute UEDVT, we recommend against the routine use of catheter extraction, surgical thrombectomy, transluminal angioplasty, stent placement, staged approach of lysis followed by interventional or surgical procedure or superior vena caval filter placement **(Grade 1C)**.
2. In selected patients with acute UEDVT (eg, those with primary UEDVT and failure of anticoagulant or thrombolytic treatment who have severe persistent symptoms), we suggest that catheter extraction, surgical thrombectomy, transluminal angioplasty, or a staged approach of lysis followed by a vascular interventional or surgical procedure may be used, if appropriate expertise and resources are available **(all Grade 2C)**.
3. In selected patients with acute UEDVT (eg, those in whom anticoagulant treatment is contraindicated and there is clear evidence of DVT progression or clinically significant PE), we suggest placement of a superior vena caval filter **(Grade 2C)**.

Anticoagulants for the Long-term Treatment of UEDVT

1. For patients with acute UEDVT, we recommend treatment with VKA for 3 months or longer **(Grade 1C)**.
   Remark: A similar process as for lower extremity DVT should be used to determine the optimal duration of anticoagulation.

2. For most patients with UEDVT in association with an indwelling central venous catheter, we suggest that the catheter not be removed if it is functional and there is an ongoing need for the catheter **(Grade 2C)**.
3. For patients who have UEDVT in association with an indwelling central venous catheter that is removed, we recommend that the duration of long-term anticoagulant treatment not be shortened to less than 3 months **(Grade 2C)**.

Prevention of Post-thrombotic Syndrome of the Arm
1. For patients at risk for post-thrombotic syndrome after UEDVT, we do not suggest routine use of elastic compression or venoactive medications **(Grade 2C)**.

Treatment of Post-thrombotic Syndrome of the Arm
1. In patients with UEDVT who have persistent edema and pain, we suggest elastic bandages or elastic compression sleeves to reduce symptoms of PTS of the upper extremity **(Grade 2C)**.

11 ANTITHROMBOTIC THERAPY IN ATRIAL FIBRILLATION

Atrial fibrillation (AF) is a common cardiac rhythm disorder, affecting nearly 2.5 million people in the United States with a lifetime risk of about 25%. Its prevalence is strongly dependent on age. It is uncommon under the age of 50, occurs at a median age of 72, and is more prevalent in men than in women at all ages.

AF is an important independent risk factor for ischemic stroke. Strokes associated with AF are thought to be cardioembolic. The rate of ischemic stroke among patients with AF is about 4.5% per year, and AF accounts for about 15% of all strokes in the United States.

EFFICACY OF ORAL ANTICOAGULANT THERAPY

Vitamin K antagonists (VKAs) are highly effective in reducing stroke in patients with atrial fibrillation. Results of clinical trials (based on intention-to-treat analysis) and from meta-analysis of five primary prevention trials and of individual-subject meta-analyses indicate that VKAs reduce the annual stroke rate from 4.5% in control patients to 1.4% for the patients assigned to adjusted-dose VKA [relative risk reduction (RRR) of 68%; 95% CI: 50 to 79%], number needed to treat (NNT)=32]. VKA treatment lowered the all-cause mortality rate by 33% (95% CI: 9 to 51%) and the combined outcome of stroke, systemic embolism, and death by 48%. Most strokes in patients assigned VKA occurred in those who had either stopped warfarin or who had subtherapeutic INR values.

VKA treatment also reduced the risk of recurrent stroke in patients with a transient ischemic attack (TIA) or minor stroke within the previous 3 months; the annual rate of stroke was reduced from 12% in control patients to 4% in anticoagulated patients (risk reduction 66%).

Pooled analysis of the first five primary prevention trials reported an annual rate of major bleeding of 1.0% in control patients compared to 1.3% in warfarin-treated patients. None of the randomized trials reported a statistically significant increase in major bleeding events in patients treated with adjusted-dose VKA.

The annual rate of intracranial hemorrhage was 0.1% in controls, compared to 0.3% in VKA users. The risk of intracranial hemorrhage increases with age, with an INR above 4.0, and in patients with associated cerebrovascular disease

EFFICACY OF ASPIRIN VERSUS PLACEBO

The results of trials with aspirin have been less consistent than those with warfarin. The most recent meta-analysis found a relative risk reduction of 24% (CI −33% to +66%) with aspirin, but the evidence of aspirin efficacy comes mainly from one trial, Stroke Prevention in Atrial Fibrillation (SPAF) I, in which a statistically significant 42% relative risk reduction was reported.

EFFICACY OF VITAMIN K ANTAGONIST VERSUS ASPIRIN

Seven trials compared VKAs with aspirin. Meta-analysis of these studies showed a 36% reduction (95% CI: 14 to 52%) in the risk of all stroke and a 46% reduction (95% CI: 27 to 60%) in the risk of ischemic stroke with adjusted-dose VKA therapy compared with aspirin. A patient-level meta-analysis from the Atrial Fibrillation Aspirin and Anticoagulation (AFASAK 1 and 2), European Atrial Fibrillation Trial (EAFT), Primary Prevention of Arterial Thromboembolism in Nonrheumatic AF in Primary Care Trial (PATAF), and SPAF II and III studies, found a relative risk reduction of 46% (95% CI: 29 to 57%) for all stroke and 52% (95% CI: 37 to 63%) for ischemic stroke with VKA compared to aspirin. Major hemorrhage was increased 1.7-fold (95% CI, for a hazard ratio of 1.21 to 2.41) with VKA.

Two trials in elderly patients also reported that VKA therapy (INR 2.0 to 3.0) was more effective than aspirin without any difference in major bleeding.

The Atrial Fibrillation Clopidogrel Trial with Irbesartan for Prevention of Vascular Events – Warfarin (ACTIVE-W) trial, which compared VKAs (INR 2.0 to 3.0) with a combination of aspirin and clopidogrel, found that VKAs reduced the risk of ischemic stroke by 53% compared with the combined antiplatelet treatment.

TRIALS COMPARING STANDARD VERSUS LOW-DOSE ANTICOAGULATION

VKA therapy targeted at INR levels of 1.5 or less is ineffective, as is fixed-dose low-intensity warfarin.

TRIALS ASSESSING A VITAMIN K ANTAGONIST COMBINED WITH AN ANTIPLATELET AGENT

Combinations of very low intensities of anticoagulation with aspirin are not effective in preventing strokes. There is, however, some evidence that combination therapy of VKA and aspirin might be effective if the targeted INR levels are below, but close to, the standard range of 2.0 to 3.0.

RISK STRATIFICATION IN PATIENTS WITH ATRIAL FIBRILLATION

Various approaches to risk stratification have been proposed. The Atrial Fibrillation Investigators (AFI) group classified patients with AF into either high- or low-risk groups for stroke. Patients were defined as high risk if they had any of the following characteristics: prior stroke or TIA, age ≥ 65 years, history of hypertension, or diabetes. Low risk was defined as the absence of these characteristics.

The SPAF investigators classified patients into three groups: high, moderate, and low risk of stroke. Patients qualified as high-risk if they had any of the following characteristics: prior stroke or TIA; women > 75 years; age > 75 years with a history of hypertension; or systolic blood pressure > 160 mm Hg (at any age). Patients were classified as moderate-risk if they had any of the following characteristics: history of hypertension, age ≤ 75 years, or diabetes. Patients were classified as low risk if they had no high- or moderate-risk features.

The CHADS$_2$ risk index uses a point system in which two points are given for a history of stroke or TIA, and one point each for age ≥ 75 years, a history of hypertension, diabetes, or recent congestive heart failure.

ANTITHROMBOTIC THERAPY FOR CHRONIC ATRIAL FLUTTER

The role of anticoagulant therapy for patients with atrial flutter has not been evaluated in clinical trials, but since these patients are at increased risk of developing AF, it is reasonable to base decisions regarding antithrombotic therapy on the risk stratification schemes used for AF.

VALVULAR HEART DISEASE AND ATRIAL FIBRILLATION

Although most randomized trials in atrial fibrillation excluded patients with valvular heart disease, the results of randomized trials in patients without valvular diseases can be generalized to patients with valvular disease, including those with prosthetic heart valves.

ATRIAL FIBRILLATION FOLLOWING CARDIAC SURGERY

Atrial fibrillation occurs in 20 to 50% of patients following open-heart surgery, usually within the first 5 days of surgery, and most commonly in the elderly.

The risk of ischemic stroke associated with postoperative AF is between 1 to 6% and is even higher among patients ≥ 75 years of age undergoing CABG surgery.

When AF persists ≥ 48 hours in the postoperative period following CABG surgery, it is appropriate to use anticoagulant therapy, although such treatment is associated with an increased risk of bleeding.

ANTICOAGULATION FOR ELECTIVE CARDIOVERSION

Evidence favoring the use of anticoagulation to prevent thromboembolism during and after cardioversion is based on observational studies and largely on electrical cardioversion. Most episodes of thromboembolism occur during the first 72 hours and are thought to be caused by migration of thrombi present within the left atrium at the time of cardioversion. The duration of anticoagulation before and after cardioversion is uncertain, but it is standard to recommend 3 weeks of prophylactic adjusted-dose warfarin (INR: 2.0 to 3.0) before, and 4 weeks after, cardioversion.

Results from several studies suggest that rates of thromboembolism are low and similar to standard warfarin therapy if transesophageal echocardiography (TEE) is used before cardioversion to detect left atrial thrombosis.

EMERGENCY CARDIOVERSION OF ATRIAL FIBRILLATION

Although studies have not been performed, treatment with heparin or low-molecular-weight heparin (LMWH) therapy at the time of cardioversion followed by anticoagulation for 4 weeks with warfarin (INR: 2.0 to 3.0) may be useful to prevent thromboembolism.

RATE VERSUS RHYTHM CONTROL IN ATRIAL FIBRILLATION

Results of recent trials indicate that high-risk patients in whom normal sinus rhythm is restored by drug treatment still require chronic warfarin anticoagulation.

RECOMMENDATIONS

Atrial Fibrillation

1. In patients with atrial fibrillation, including those with paroxysmal atrial fibrillation, who have had a prior ischemic stroke, transient ischemic attack, or systemic embolism, we recommend long-term anticoagulation with an oral vitamin K antagonist, such as warfarin, targeted at an INR of 2.5 (range: 2.0 to 3.0) because of the high risk of future ischemic stroke faced by this set of patients **(Grade 1A)**. Timing of the initiation of VKA therapy after an acute ischemic stroke involves balancing the risk of hemorrhagic conversion with short-term risk of recurrent ischemic stroke and is addressed in Chapter 13, Antithrombotic and Thrombolytic Therapy for Ischemic Stroke.

2. In patients with atrial fibrillation, including those with paroxysmal atrial fibrillation, who have two or more of the following risk factors for future ischemic stroke, we recommend long-term anticoagulation with an oral vitamin K antagonist, such as warfarin, targeted at an INR of 2.5 (range: 2.0 to 3.0) because of the increased risk of future ischemic stroke faced by this set of patients **(Grade 1A)**.

   Two or more of the following risk factors apply:
   - age > 75 years
   - history of hypertension
   - diabetes mellitus
   - moderately or severely impaired left ventricular systolic function and/or heart failure

3. In patients with atrial fibrillation, including those with paroxysmal AF, with only one of the risk factors listed below, we recommend long-term antithrombotic therapy **(Grade 1A)**, either as anticoagulation with an oral vitamin K antagonist, such as warfarin, targeted at an INR

of 2.5 (range: 2.0 to 3.0) **(Grade 1A)**, or as aspirin, at a dose of 75 to 325 mg/d **(Grade 1B)**. For these patients at intermediate risk of ischemic stroke, we suggest a VKA rather than aspirin **(Grade 2A)**. This set of patients with atrial fibrillation is defined by having one of the following risk factors:

- age > 75 years
- history of hypertension
- diabetes mellitus
- moderately or severely impaired left ventricular systolic function and/or heart failure

4. In patients with atrial fibrillation, including those with paroxysmal AF, aged ≤ 75 years and with none of the other risk factors listed above, we recommend long-term aspirin therapy at a dose of 75 to 325 mg/d **(Grade 1B)** because of their low risk of ischemic stroke.

Remarks: (1) These recommendations apply to patients with persistent or paroxysmal AF and not to patients with a single brief episode of AF due to a reversible cause, such as an acute pulmonary infection. (2) The optimal dose of aspirin for patients with AF is unclear. The largest effect of aspirin was seen in the first Stroke Prevention in AF (SPAF I) trial, which used aspirin at 325 mg/d. However, generalizing from trials of aspirin for all antithrombotic indications and from physiologic studies, we feel the best balance of efficacy and safety is achieved at low doses of aspirin (ie, 75 to 100 mg/d).

Atrial Flutter

1. For patients with atrial flutter, we recommend that antithrombotic therapy decisions follow the same risk-based recommendations as for AF **(Grade 1C)**.

Valvular Heart Disease and Atrial Fibrillation

1. For patients with AF and mitral stenosis, we recommend long-term anticoagulation with an oral vitamin K antagonist, such as warfarin (target INR: 2.5; range: 2.0 to 3.0) **(Grade 1B)**.

2. For patients with AF and prosthetic heart valves, we recommend long-term anticoagulation with an oral vitamin K antagonist, such as warfarin, at a dose intensity appropriate for the specific type of prosthesis **(Grade 1B)**. See Chapter 12, Valvular and Structural Heart Disease, for antithrombotic management of patients with valvular heart disease and AF.

Atrial Fibrillation Following Cardiac Surgery

1. For patients with AF occurring shortly after open-heart surgery and lasting 48 hours or more, we suggest anticoagulation with an oral VKA,

such as warfarin, if bleeding risks are acceptable **(Grade 2C)**. The target INR is 2.5 (range: 2.0 to 3.0). We suggest continuing anticoagulation for 4 weeks following reversion to, and maintenance of, normal sinus rhythm (NSR), particularly if patients have risk factors for thromboembolism **(Grade 2C)**.

Anticoagulation for Elective Cardioversion of Atrial Fibrillation

1. For patients with AF of 48 hours or longer or of unknown duration, for whom pharmacologic or electrical cardioversion is planned, we recommend anticoagulation with an oral vitamin K antagonist, such as warfarin, at a target INR of 2.5 (range: 2.0 to 3.0) for 3 weeks before elective cardioversion and for at least 4 weeks after sinus rhythm has been maintained **(Grade 1C)**.

   Remark: This recommendation applies to all patients with atrial fibrillation, including those whose risk factor status would otherwise indicate a low risk for stroke. Patients with risk factors for thromboembolism should continue anticoagulation beyond 4 weeks unless there is convincing evidence that sinus rhythm is maintained. For patients with recurrent episodes of AF, see 1, 2, 3, and 4 under "Atrial Fibrillation" above.

2. For patients with AF of 48 hours or longer, or of unknown duration, who are undergoing pharmacologic or electrical cardioversion, we recommend either immediate anticoagulation with intravenous (IV) unfractionated heparin (target activated partial thromboplastin time [APTT] 60 s; range: 50 to 70 s), or low-molecular-weight heparin (at full deep venous thrombosis [DVT] treatment doses), or at least 5 days of warfarin (target INR of 2.5; range: 2.0 to 3.0) at the time of cardioversion and performance of a screening multiplane TEE. If no thrombus is seen, cardioversion is successful, and sinus rhythm is maintained, we recommend anticoagulation (target INR: 2.5; range: 2.0 to 3.0) for at least 4 weeks. If a thrombus is seen on TEE, then cardioversion should be postponed and anticoagulation should be continued indefinitely. We recommend obtaining a repeat TEE before attempting later cardioversion (all **Grade 1B** addressing the equivalence of TEE-guided versus non-TEE-guided cardioversion).

   Remark: The utility of the conventional and TEE-guided approaches is likely comparable. This recommendation applies to all patients with atrial fibrillation, including those whose risk factor status would otherwise indicate a low risk for stroke. Patients with risk factors for thromboembolism should continue anticoagulation beyond 4 weeks unless there is convincing evidence that sinus rhythm is maintained. For patients with recurrent episodes of AF, see "Atrial Fibrillation" above.

3. For patients with AF of known duration of < 48 hours, we suggest that cardioversion be performed without prolonged anticoagulation **(Grade 2C)**. However, in patients without contraindications to anticoagulation, we suggest beginning IV heparin (target PTT: 60 s; range: 50 to 70 s) or LMWH (at full DVT treatment doses) at presentation **(Grade 2C)**.

   Remark: For patients with risk factors for stroke, it is particularly important to be confident that the duration of AF is < 48 hours. In such patients with risk factors, a TEE-guided approach is a reasonable alternative strategy. Postcardioversion anticoagulation is based on whether the patient has experienced more than one episode of AF, and on his or her risk-factor status. For patients with recurrent episodes of AF, see "Atrial Fibrillation" above.

4. For emergency cardioversion in the hemodynamically unstable patient, we suggest that IV unfractionated heparin (target PTT of 60 s with a target range of 50 to 70 s) or low-molecular-weight heparin (at full DVT treatment doses) be started as soon as possible, followed by at least 4 weeks of anticoagulation with an oral vitamin K antagonist, such as warfarin (target INR of 2.5; range: 2.0 to 3.0) if cardioversion is successful and sinus rhythm is maintained **(Grade 2C)**.

   Remark: Long-term continuation of anticoagulation is based on whether the patient has experienced more than one episode of AF and on his or her risk-factor status. For patients experiencing more than one episode of AF, see "Atrial Fibrillation" above.

5. For cardioversion of patients with atrial flutter, we suggest use of anticoagulants in the same way as for cardioversion of patients with atrial fibrillation **(Grade 2C)**.

12 VALVULAR AND STRUCTURAL HEART DISEASE

RHEUMATIC MITRAL VALVE DISEASE (MITRAL STENOSIS AND/OR MITRAL REGURGITATION)

The risk of systemic embolism is greater in rheumatic mitral valve disease than in any other common form of valvular heart disease, and is increased further with the development of atrial fibrillation (AF). The risk of thromboembolism also increases with age. Other risk factors for systemic embolism include the presence of a left atrial thrombus, low cardiac output, and significant aortic regurgitation. Mitral valvuloplasty does not appear to eliminate the risk of thromboembolism, although it might reduce it.

Patients who suffer a first embolus are at high risk of recurrent embolism. This risk is not eliminated by mitral valvuloplasty. Thus, a successful mitral valvuloplasty does not eliminate the need for anticoagulation in patients who required long-term anticoagulation prior to the procedure.

Although never evaluated by randomized trial, there is a strong impression that long-term anticoagulant therapy is effective in reducing the incidence of systemic emboli in patients with rheumatic mitral valve disease and AF, but there is uncertainty about the need to use long-term anticoagulation in patients with mitral stenosis who are in sinus rhythm.

Percutaneous balloon mitral valvuloplasty is commonly used to treat mitral stenosis. Transesophageal echocardiography (TEE) can be performed prior to balloon mitral valvuloplasty, and if there is no left atrial thrombus, anticoagulation prior to the valvuloplasty can be avoided. If a left atrial thrombus is present, the procedure should be postponed and the patient treated with anticoagulants.

MITRAL VALVE PROLAPSE

Mitral valve prolapse (MVP) is the most common form of valve disease in adults. About 6% of the female and 4% of the male population have MVP. The risk of stroke in young adults with MVP is very low (only 1/6,000 per year). Long-term warfarin therapy is appropriate for those patients with AF and for those who continue to have cerebral ischemic events despite aspirin therapy.

MITRAL ANNULAR CALCIFICATION

Mitral annular calcification (MAC) can be associated with mitral stenosis and regurgitation, calcific aortic stenosis, conduction disturbances, arrhythmias, embolic complications, and endocarditis. Emboli can arise from thrombi on the calcific valve or they can be composed of calcified spicules. Most patients are elderly (mean age: 74 years).

MAC is an independent risk factor for stroke, and the prevalence of AF is 12 times greater in patients with MAC than in those without. Clinical trials with antithrombotic therapy have not been reported.

AORTIC VALVE AND AORTIC ARCH DISORDERS

Clinically detectable systemic emboli are uncommon in isolated aortic valve disease (stenosis or sclerosis). Small calcific microemboli are not rare, but usually do not produce clinical symptoms.

Patients with atherosclerotic plaques of the aortic arch and ascending aorta detected by TEE have an increased risk of ischemic stroke. Mobile aortic plaques or plaques greater than, or equal to, 4 mm in thickness are associated with an increased risk of vascular events; this risk is further increased by a lack of plaque calcification.

PATENT FORAMEN OVALE (PFO) AND ATRIAL SEPTAL ANEURYSM

Patent foramen ovale (PFO) is observed at autopsy in about 28% of otherwise normal hearts. Paradoxical embolism through a PFO is well documented, as is thrombus on the arterial side of an atrial septal aneurysm. However, the importance of these conditions as causes of stroke remains uncertain, as does the indication for anticoagulants.

Patients with unexplained cerebral ischemia or stroke who have right-to-left shunting through a PFO should be investigated for the presence of deep venous thrombosis (DVT). If DVT is found, such patients should be considered for either long-term anticoagulation or closure of the septal defect.

MECHANICAL AND BIOPROSTHETIC VALVES

Patients with prosthetic heart valve replacements are at risk of systemic embolism. The risk of systemic embolism is greater with mechanical rather than bioprosthetic valves, with prosthetic mitral rather than aortic valves, and if there is associated AF. In addition, the newer mechanical valves appear to be less thrombogenic than older valves. For patients with tissue prosthetic valves who are in sinus rhythm, the risk of embolism is thought to be largely confined to the first 3 months after valve insertion. In contrast, the risk is life-long in patients with mechanical prosthetic valves (particularly in the mitral position).

MECHANICAL PROSTHETIC VALVES

Randomized trials have shown that warfarin is effective in reducing the risk of systemic embolism in patients with mechanical prosthetic valves when given at a lower intensity than has been used in the past. A targeted INR of 2.0 to 3.0 appears satisfactory for patients with St. Jude bileaflet and Medtronic-Hall tilting disc mechanical valves in the aortic position, provided they are in sinus rhythm and the left atrium is not enlarged, whereas a targeted INR of 2.5 to 3.5 is suggested for tilting disc valves and bileaflet prosthetic valves in the mitral position. The addition of aspirin to warfarin reduces the risk of stroke and vascular death, compared with warfarin alone, but at a cost of an increased risk of bleeding. If embolic complications occur at the recommended INR intensity, then either aspirin 80 mg/d or dipyridamole 300 mg/d should be added to warfarin, since both antiplatelet agents augment the efficacy of warfarin when used for this indication.

BIOPROSTHETIC VALVES

The risk of thromboembolism is less with uncomplicated bioprosthetic valves than with mechanical valves. Warfarin is just as effective, but much safer, when used at a targeted INR of 2.0 to 3.0 than when used at an INR of 3.0 to 4.5. Consequently, the less intense therapeutic range of 2.0 to 3.0 is indicated. Although the risk of thromboembolism may be limited mainly to the first 3 months postoperatively in the uncomplicated patient, it is present indefinitely if there is associated AF. The risk of systemic embolism is less in patients with aortic bioprosthetic valves, so the case for oral anticoagulants is less compelling. Longer-term anticoagulant therapy is indicated in patients with AF and in those with an atrial thrombus detected at echocardiography.

INFECTIVE ENDOCARDITIS

Patients with infective endocarditis are at high risk for systemic embolism, but the use of anticoagulants in these patients is problematic because they are also at high risk of intracranial bleeding. Embolic risk increases in the following circumstances: (1) in acute endocarditis versus subacute endocarditis, (2) in mitral valve endocarditis versus aortic valve endocarditis, and (3) in mechanical prosthetic valve endocarditis versus native valve or bioprosthetic valve endocarditis.

   In general, anticoagulants are not indicated in patients with native valve or bioprosthetic valve endocarditis because the risk of intracranial bleeding is thought to outweigh the benefits of treatment. However, in the higher risk mechanical bioprosthetic valve endocarditis, discontinuation of anticoagulant therapy is not recommended because the risk of cerebral embolism in untreated patients is thought to be greater than the risk of intracranial hemorrhage.

NONBACTERIAL THROMBOTIC ENDOCARDITIS

Nonbacterial thrombotic endocarditis (NBTE) occurs in patients with malignancies, in patients with other chronic debilitating diseases, and in patients with acute fulminant diseases, such as septicemia, or burns. Systemic embolism occurs in about 40% of patients with NBTE. The diagnosis of NBTE is difficult. Cardiac murmurs are often absent, and echocardiography is less sensitive for the detection of NBTE than it is for bacterial endocarditis. Heparin appears to be effective in preventing embolic events in these patients, whereas limited data suggest that warfarin is ineffective.

RECOMMENDATIONS

1. For patients with rheumatic mitral valve disease, complicated singly or in combination by the presence of AF, previous systemic embolism, or left atrial thrombus, we recommend vitamin K antagonist (VKA) therapy (target INR: 2.5; range: 2.0 to 3.0) **(Grade 1A)**.

2. For patients with rheumatic mitral valve disease with AF who suffer systemic embolism or develop left atrial thrombus while receiving VKAs at a therapeutic INR, we suggest the addition of low-dose acetylsalicylic acid (ASA, or aspirin) therapy (50 to 100 mg/d) after consideration of the additional hemorrhagic risk **(Grade 2C)**. An alternative strategy might be the adjustment of VKA dosing to achieve a higher target INR (target INR: 3.0; range: 2.5 to 3.5) **(Grade 2C)**.

3. In patients with rheumatic mitral valve disease and normal sinus rhythm with a left atrial diameter < 55 mm, we do not suggest antithrombotic therapy unless a separate indication exists **(Grade 2C)**.

4. For patients being considered for PMBV, we recommend a pre-procedural TEE to exclude left atrial thrombus **(Grade 1C)**.

5. For patients being considered for percutaneous mitral balloon angioplasty (PMBV) with pre-procedural TEE showing left atrial thrombus, we recommend postponement of PMBV and VKA therapy (target INR: 3.0; range: 2.5 to 3.5) until thrombus resolution is documented by repeat TEE **(Grade 1C)**. If left atrial thrombus does not resolve with VKA therapy, we recommend that PMBV not be performed **(Grade 1C)**.

6. In patients with MVP who have not experienced systemic embolism, unexplained transient ischemic attack (TIA) or ischemic stroke, and who do not have AF, we recommend against any antithrombotic therapy **(Grade 1C)**.

7. In patients with MVP who have documented but unexplained TIAs or ischemic stroke, we recommend ASA therapy (50 to 100 mg/d) **(Grade 1B)**.

8. In patients with MVP who have documented systemic embolism or recurrent TIAs despite ASA therapy, we suggest VKA therapy (target INR: 2.5; range: 2.0 to 3.0) **(Grade 2C)**.

9. In patients with MAC complicated by systemic embolism, ischemic stroke, or TIA, who do not have AF, we recommend ASA (50 to 100 mg/d) **(Grade 1B)**. For recurrent events despite ASA therapy, we suggest that treatment with VKA therapy might be considered (target INR: 2.5; range: 2.0 to 3.0) **(Grade 2C)**. In patients with MAC who have a single embolus documented to be calcific, the data is not sufficient to allow recommendation for or against antithrombotic therapy.

10. In patients with MAC and AF we recommend VKA therapy (target INR: 2.5; range: 2.0 to 3.0) **(Grade 1C)**.

11. In patients with isolated calcific aortic valve disease who have not experienced ischemic stroke or TIA, we recommend against antithrombotic therapy **(Grade 2C)**.

12. In patients with isolated calcific aortic valve disease who have experienced ischemic stroke or TIA not attributable to another source, we suggest ASA (50 to 100 mg/d) **(Grade 2C)**.

13. In patients with ischemic stroke associated with aortic atherosclerotic lesions, we recommend low-dose ASA (50 to 100 mg/d) over no therapy **(Grade 1C)**. For patients with ischemic stroke associated with mobile aortic arch thrombi, we suggest therapy with either VKAs (target INR: 2.5; range: 2.0 to 3.0) or low-dose ASA (50 to 100 mg/d) **(Grade 2C)**.

14. In patients with ischemic stroke and a PFO, we recommend antiplatelet (AP) therapy **(Grade 1A)**, and suggest AP therapy over VKA therapy **(Grade 2A)**.

15. In patients with cryptogenic ischemic stroke and PFO, with evidence of DVT or another indication for VKA therapy, such as AF or an underlying hypercoagulable state, we recommend VKA therapy (target INR: 2.5; range: 2.0 to 3.0) **(Grade 1C)**.

16. In patients with mechanical heart valves, we recommend VKA therapy **(Grade 1A)**. Immediately following mechanical valve replacement, and as dictated by clinical concerns regarding postoperative bleeding, we suggest administration of intravenous UFH or subcutaneous LMWH until the INR is stable and at a therapeutic level for 2 consecutive days **(Grade 2C)**.

17. In patients with a bileaflet mechanical valve or a Medtronic Hall tilting disk valve in the aortic position, who are in sinus rhythm and without left atrial enlargement, we recommend VKA therapy (target INR: 2.5; range: 2.0 to 3.0) **(Grade 1B)**.

18. In patients with a tilting disk or bileaflet mechanical valve in the mitral position, we recommend VKA therapy (target INR: 3.0; range: 2.5 to 3.5) **(Grade 1B)**.

19. In patients with a caged ball or caged disk valve, we recommend VKA therapy (target INR: 3.0; range: 2.5 to 3.5) **(Grade 1B)**.

20. In patients with mechanical heart valves in either or both the aortic or mitral position, and who have additional risk factors for thromboembolism, such as AF, anterior-apical ST-segment elevation myocardial infarction (STEMI), left atrial enlargement, hypercoagulable state, or low ejection fraction, we recommend VKA therapy (target INR: 3.0; range: 2.5 to 3.5) **(Grade 1B)**.

21. In patients with mechanical heart valves who have additional risk factors for thromboembolism, such as AF, hypercoagulable state, or low ejection fraction, or who have a history of atherosclerotic vascular disease, we recommend the addition of low-dose ASA (50 to 100 mg/d) to chronic VKA therapy **(Grade 1B)**. We suggest ASA not be added to VKA therapy in patients with mechanical heart valves who are at particularly high risk of bleeding; such as those with prior history of gastrointestinal bleed or in patients older than 80 years of age **(Grade 2C)**.

22. In patients with mechanical prosthetic heart valves who suffer systemic embolism despite a therapeutic INR, we suggest the addition of aspirin (50 to 100 mg/d) if not previously provided and/or upward titration of VKA therapy to achieve a higher target INR. For a previous target INR of 2.5, we suggest the VKA dose be increased to achieve a target INR of 3.0 (range: 2.5 to 3.5). For a previous target INR of 3.0, we suggest the VKA dose be increased to achieve a target INR of 3.5 (range: 3.0 to 4.0) **(Grade 2C)**.

23. In patients with a bioprosthetic valve in the mitral position, we recommend VKA therapy (target INR: 2.5; range: 2.0 to 3.0) for the first 3 months after valve insertion **(Grade 1B)**. In the early postoperative period, in the absence of concerns for significant bleeding, we suggest administration of intravenous unfractionated heparin (UFH) or subcutaneous low-molecular-weight heparin (LMWH) until the INR is at therapeutic levels for 2 consecutive days **(Grade 2C)**. After the first 3 months, in patients who are in sinus rhythm and have no other indication for VKA therapy, we recommend ASA (50 to 100 mg/d) **(Grade 1B)**.

24. In patients with bioprosthetic valves, who are in sinus rhythm and have no other indication for VKA therapy, we recommend long-term therapy with ASA (50 to 100 mg/d) **(Grade 1B)**.

25. In patients with bioprosthetic valves who have a prior history of systemic embolism, we recommend VKA therapy (target INR: 2.5; range: 2.0 to 3.0) for at least 3 months after valve insertion, followed by careful clinical reassessment **(Grade 1C)**.

26. In patients with bioprosthetic valves who have evidence of a left atrial thrombus at surgery, we recommend VKA therapy (target INR: 2.5; range: 2.0 to 3.0) until documented thrombus resolution **(Grade 1C)**.

27. In patients with bioprosthetic valves who have additional risk factors for thromboembolism, including AF, hypercoagulable state, or low ejection fraction, we recommend VKA therapy (target INR: 2.5; range: 2.0 to 3.0) **(Grade 1C)**. We suggest the addition of low-dose aspirin (50 to 100 mg/d) be considered, particularly in patients with a history of atherosclerotic vascular disease **(Grade 2C)**. We suggest ASA not be added to chronic VKA therapy in patients with bioprosthetic heart valves who are at particularly high risk of bleeding, such as patients with a prior history of gastrointestinal bleeding or in patients older than 80 years of age **(Grade 2C)**.

28. For patients with right-sided prosthetic valve thrombosis (PVT), with large thrombus size, or New York Heart Association (NYHA) functional class III to IV, we recommend administration of fibrinolytic therapy **(Grade 1C)**.

29. For patients with left-sided PVT, NYHA functional class I to II, and small thrombus area (< 0.8 cm^2), we suggest administration of fibrinolytic therapy. Alternatively, administration of intravenous UFH, accompanied by serial Doppler echocardiography to document thrombus resolution or improvement, can be considered for very small, nonobstructive thrombus **(Grade 2C)**.

30. For patients with left-sided PVT, NYHA functional class III to IV, and small thrombus area (< 0.8 cm^2), we suggest fibrinolytic therapy **(Grade 2C)**.

31. For patients with left-sided PVT and large thrombus area (≥ 0.8 cm^2), we suggest emergency surgery be considered. If surgery is not available or considered high risk, we suggest fibrinolytic therapy **(Grade 2C)**.

32. For patients who have had successful resolution of PVT, we suggest initiation of intravenous UFH and VKA therapy. We suggest intravenous UFH be continued until a therapeutic INR is achieved. For a mechanical valve in the aortic position, we suggest maintaining a higher INR (target: 3.5; range: 3.0 to 4.0) plus ASA (50 to 100 mg/d).

33. For a mechanical valve in the mitral position, we suggest maintaining a higher INR (target: 4.0; range: 3.5 to 4.5) plus ASA (50 to 100 mg/d) **(Grade 2C)**.

34. In patients with infective endocarditis (IE), we recommend against routine antithrombotic therapy, unless a separate, strong indication exists **(Grade 1B)**.

35. In the patient treated with VKA therapy who develops IE, we suggest VKA be discontinued at the time of initial presentation and UFH sub-

stituted until it is clear that invasive procedures will not be required, and the patient has stabilized without signs of central nervous system (CNS) involvement. When the patient is deemed stable without contraindications or neurologic complications, we suggest reinstitution of long-term VKA therapy **(Grade 2C)**.

36. In patients with NBTE and systemic or pulmonary emboli, we recommend treatment with full-dose IV UFH or subcutaneous LMWH **(Grade 1C)**.

37. In patients with disseminated cancer or debilitating disease with aseptic vegetations, we suggest administration of full-dose IV UFH or subcutaneous LMWH **(Grade 2C)**.

13 ANTITHROMBOTIC AND THROMBOLYTIC THERAPY FOR ISCHEMIC STROKE

Optimal antithrombotic treatment of ischemic stroke requires knowledge of the cause of stroke, which can sometimes be difficult to determine with certainty. About 30% of ischemic strokes remain cryptogenic after extensive investigation. Atherosclerosis of both small and large arteries supplying the brain is the most common cause of ischemic stroke. About 20% of ischemic strokes are due to cardiogenic embolism, most commonly from atrial fibrillation (AF). Lipohyalinosis and other occlusive diseases of the small penetrating brain arteries are the most frequent causes of small, subcortical lacunar infarcts.

Strokes caused by large-artery atherosclerosis have the worst prognosis, and lacunar strokes have the best prognosis. The risk of early recurrence in patients with cardioembolic strokes is related to the underlying cardiac lesion.

Cardiogenic embolism occurs in association with atrial fibrillation, mitral stenosis, mechanical prosthetic valves, recent myocardial infarction (MI), left ventricular mural thrombus, atrial myxoma, dilated cardiomyopathies, infective endocarditis, and marantic endocarditis. The occurrence of multiple infarctions in different vascular territories or the history of systemic emboli increases the likelihood of a cardiac embolism as the cause of stroke.

Cryptogenic infarcts are thought to be cardioembolic, although other causes, such as paradoxical emboli through a patent foramen ovale (PFO), unrecognized arterial lesions (dissections, mild atherosclerosis), or aortic arch atherosclerosis have to be considered.

TREATMENT OF ISCHEMIC STROKE

Thrombolytic therapy and antithrombotic therapy are effective in selected patients with stroke. Most stroke patients are not eligible for intravenous (IV) recombinant tissue plasminogen activator (rt-PA) therapy and are treated with antithrombotic agents.

Thrombolytic Therapy

Despite increasing the early rate of intracranial hemorrhage, IV tissue plasminogen activator (t-PA) improves functional outcome at 3 months when administered to selected patients within 3 hours of acute ischemic stroke onset. The risk of cerebral hemorrhage is increased by the severity of neurologic deficit, the presence of brain edema, or mass effect on the pretreatment computed tomography (CT) scan, and by uncontrolled hypertension. In contrast to results with t-PA, the use of streptokinase is associated with an increased incidence of adverse outcomes (mortality and cerebral hemorrhage). Regulatory approval for t-PA use in stroke has been issued in the United States, Canada, Europe, Australia, and other countries.

Results of randomized studies with intra-arterial thrombolytic therapy recombinant pro-urokinase (rpro-UK) were equivocal when the thrombolytic agent was administered within less than 6 hours of stroke caused by middle cerebral arterial thrombosis. However, results from several case studies using intra-arterial thrombolysis in patients with acute basilar artery thrombosis (without controls) suggested the possibility of benefit.

Antithrombotic Agents (Heparin, Low-Molecular-Weight Heparin, Heparinoid and Antiplatelet Agents)

A variety of antithrombotic agents, including heparin, low-molecular-weight heparins (LMWHs), and heparinoids and aspirin [acetylsalicylic acid (ASA)] have been evaluated for acute cerebral infarction patients who are not eligible for thrombolytic therapy. In general, the results with anticoagulants have been disappointing, whereas those with aspirin have been more promising.

Immediate anticoagulation of patients with acute ischemic stroke does not appear to reduce death or dependency.

The results in the heparin arm of the large international stroke study suggest that the use of early unmonitored high-dose subcutaneous heparin reduces early stroke recurrence risks but at the cost of increased hemorrhagic complications. The use of lower doses of heparin may reduce the hemorrhagic side effects and may retain some benefits.

Neither LMWH nor danaparoid was shown to be effective in stroke patients in recent trials.

Cardioembolic Stroke

Oral anticoagulants substantially reduce the long-term risk of cardiac embolism, but the evidence supporting early anticoagulation in acute cardioembolic stroke is inconclusive and the risk of symptomatic hemorrhagic transformation with acute anticoagulation is greater than the risk with antiplatelet therapy.

Antiplatelet Agents for Altering Outcomes in Acute Stroke in Patients Not Eligible for Thrombolysis

Aspirin is the only antiplatelet agent that has been evaluated for the treatment of acute ischemic stroke. In a meta-analysis of 41,399 subjects enrolled in nine trials, death or dependency at 6 months was significantly less for those treated with aspirin, although the benefit was small [odds ratio (OR) = 0.94; 95% confidence interval (CI): 0.91 to 0.98].

Antithrombotic Therapy for Prevention of Deep Vein Thrombosis and Pulmonary Embolism in Acute Ischemic Stroke

Deep vein thrombosis and pulmonary embolism are frequent complications of stroke, with about 5% of early deaths attributed to PE. In an overview analysis among acute stroke patients, anticoagulants were associated with four fewer pulmonary emboli per 1,000 (OR = 0.60, 95% CI: 0.44 to 0.81). Low-molecular-weight heparins are either equivalent to, or better than, unfractionated heparin (UFH) in preventing DVT.

STROKE PREVENTION

Antiplatelet Agents

Aspirin, ticlopidine, clopidogrel, and dipyridamole (particularly when combined with aspirin) are effective for prevention of stroke.

In an analysis of 144,051 patients with previous MI, acute MI, previous transient ischemic attack (TIA)/stroke, acute stroke, and other patients at increased risk of atherothrombotic events, antiplatelet agents reduced the odds of the composite outcome of stroke, MI, or vascular death by about 25%. The odds reduction attributable to aspirin alone was 23%. Antiplatelet drugs reduced the odds of a nonfatal stroke by 25%, nonfatal MI by about 34%, and vascular mortality by 15%.

For patients with prior stroke or TIA, aspirin reduced the odds for the composite outcome of stroke, MI, or vascular death by only 16%. The efficacy of aspirin appears to be independent of aspirin dose, although a recent study in patients undergoing carotid endarterectomy reported that low-dose aspirin is more effective than high-dose. Aspirin is also effective in reducing stroke in patients undergoing carotid endarterectomy.

Clopidogrel is marginally more effective than aspirin in stroke patients (relative risk reduction 8%).

Combination Antiplatelet Therapy

In stroke patients, the combination of clopidogrel plus aspirin is not more effective, and is associated with an increased risk of bleeding compared with clopidogrel monotherapy. In stroke/TIA patients, the combination of slow-release dipyridamole and aspirin produces about an 18% reduction in stroke, MI, and vascular death without a significant increase in bleeding, compared to aspirin alone.

Vitamin K Antagonists

Vitamin K antagonists are effective for both primary and secondary prevention of stroke in patients with AF and other conditions associated with cardiogenic embolism. In contrast, there is no evidence that coumarins are effective in non-cardioembolic stroke, but there is evidence that (1) when used at a targeted INR of 3.0 to 4.5, oral anticoagulant therapy causes unacceptably high rates of intracranial hemorrhage, (2) warfarin (target INR: 1.4 to 2.8) is no better than aspirin, and (3) warfarin (target INR: 2.0 to 3.0) causes more adverse outcome than aspirin in patients with symptomatic stenosis of a major intracranial artery.

PREVENTION OF CARDIOEMBOLIC CEREBRAL ISCHEMIC EVENTS

Atrial fibrillation is responsible for about 50% of all cardiogenic emboli. Other high-risk sources of cardiogenic embolism include mitral stenosis, mechanical prosthetic valves, recent MI, left ventricular mural thrombus, atrial myxoma, dilated cardiomyopathies, infective endocarditis, and marantic endocarditis.

Patients with Acute Stroke and Underlying Atrial Fibrillation: Anticoagulation

Oral anticoagulant therapy is highly effective for both primary and secondary prevention of stroke in patients with atrial fibrillation. In general, oral anticoagulation therapy is recommended within 2 weeks of a cardioembolic stroke; however, for patients with large infarcts or other risk factors for hemorrhage, additional delays may be appropriate.

Patients with Stroke with Underlying Atrial Fibrillation: Antiplatelet Agents

Two large randomized studies have evaluated the efficacy of antiplatelet agents for secondary prevention of cardiac embolism. In the first—the European Atrial Fibrillation Trial (EAFT)—aspirin (compared to untreated control) was associated with a 16% (non-significant) reduction in the relative risk of stroke (not significant [NS]). In the second—Studio Italiano Fibrillazione Atriale (SIFA)—indobufen (a reversible inhibitor of cyclooxygenase) was compared with warfarin (INR: 2.0 to 3.5) and no significant difference in the incidence of stroke, MI, PE, or vascular death was noted between the two groups.

OTHER CAUSES OF EMBOLIC STROKE

Aortic Atheromata

Complex atherosclerotic aortic plaques are an independent risk factor for embolic stroke. Plaques of greater than 4 to 5 mm in thickness, ulcerated plaques, and those with mobile components are more likely to be associated with stroke. Information on the effectiveness of antithrombotic therapy in preventing stroke associated with aortic atherosclerosis is sparse.

Patent Foramen Ovale

A patent foramen ovale (PFO) is a potential cause of cryptogenic stroke in young patients. Patients with complex PFOs (eg, the combination of a large PFO and atrial septal aneurysm) may be at higher risk for recurrent stroke, although the data are not consistent.

Mitral Valve Prolapse

Recent population-based prospective studies failed to find an increased risk of ischemic stroke associated with this common echocardiographic finding.

CEREBRAL VENOUS SINUS THROMBOSIS

Risk factors for cerebral venous sinus thrombosis (CVST) include pregnancy, estrogens, and inherited thrombophilic disorders. The risk in thrombophilia is increased further in women who are taking oral contraceptives. The prognosis of CVST is generally much better than previously thought, but remains largely unpredictable. The limited data from two small randomized studies suggest that both unfractionated and low-molecular-weight heparins are likely to be safe and effective in these patients. There is controversy regarding the benefit-to-risk ratio in patients with large hemorrhagic venous infarcts with associated hematomas.

RECOMMENDATIONS

Intravenous t-PA for Acute Ischemic Stroke Within 3 Hours of Symptom Onset

1. For eligible patients (see inclusion and exclusion criteria listed below), we recommend administration of IV t-PA in a dose of 0.9 mg/kg (maximum of 90 mg), with 10% of the total dose given as an initial bolus and the remainder infused over 60 minutes, provided that treatment is initiated within 3 hours of clearly defined symptom onset **(Grade 1A)**.

2. We recommend that patients who are eligible for t-PA be treated as quickly as possible within the 3 hour time limit **(Grade 1A)**.
   Remark: All unnecessary delays must be avoided because the benefits of t-PA therapy diminish rapidly over time.

3. For patients with extensive (greater than one-third of the middle cerebral artery territory) and clearly identifiable hypodensity on CT, we suggest not using t-PA in this situation **(Grade 2B)**.

Intravenous t-PA for Acute Ischemic Stroke Between 3 Hours to 6 Hours of Symptom Onset

1. For patients with acute ischemic stroke of greater than 3 hours but less than 4.5 hours, we suggest clinicians do not use intravenous t-PA **(Grade 2A)**. For patients with acute stroke onset of greater than 4.5 hours, we recommend against the use of intravenous t-PA **(Grade 1A)**.

Intravenous Streptokinase for Acute Ischemic Stroke Between 0 and 6 hours of Symptom Onset

1. For patients with acute ischemic stroke, we recommend against streptokinase **(Grade 1A)**.

Intra-Arterial Thrombolysis for Acute Ischemic Stroke

1. For patients with angiographically demonstrated middle cerebral artery (MCA) occlusion and without signs of major early infarct on the baseline CT or magnetic resonance imaging (MRI) scan, who can be treated within 6 hours of symptom onset, we suggest intra-arterial thrombolytic therapy with t-PA for selected patients in centers with the appropriate neurologic and interventional expertise **(Grade 2C)**.

2. For patients with acute basilar artery thrombosis and without major CT/MRI evidence of infarction, we suggest either intra-arterial or intravenous thrombolysis with t-PA depending on available resources and capabilities **(Grade 2C)**.

Anticoagulants for Altering Outcomes Among Acute Stroke in Patients Not Eligible For Thrombolysis

1. For patients with acute ischemic stroke, we recommend against full-dose anticoagulation with intravenous, subcutaneous, or low-molecular-weight heparins or heparinoids **(Grade 1B)**.

Antiplatelet Agents for Altering Outcomes in Acute Stroke Patients Not Eligible For Thrombolysis

1. For patients with acute ischemic stroke who are not receiving thrombolysis, we recommend early aspirin therapy (initial dose of 150 to 325 mg) **(Grade 1A)**.

Antithrombotic Therapy for Prevention of DVT and PE in Acute Ischemic Stroke

1. For acute stroke patients with restricted mobility, we recommend prophylactic low-dose subcutaneous heparin or low-molecular-weight heparins **(Grade 1A)**.
2. For patients who have contraindications to anticoagulants, use of intermittent pneumatic compression devices or elastic stockings **(Grade 1B)**.

Intermittent Pneumatic Compression DVT/PE Prophylaxis in Patients With Intracerebral Hematoma

1. In patients with an acute intracerebral hematoma, we recommend the initial use of intermittent pneumatic compression devices **(Grade 1B)**.

Heparin for DVT/PE Prophylaxis in Patients With Intracerebral Hematoma

1. In stable patients, we suggest low-dose subcutaneous heparin as soon as the second day after the onset of the hemorrhage **(Grade 2C)**.

Prevention of Cerebral Ischemic Events in Patients With Non-Cardioembolic TIA or Stroke: Antiplatelet Drugs Versus Placebo or Versus an Alternative Antiplatelet Drug

1. In patients who have experienced a non-cardioembolic stroke or TIA (ie, atherothrombotic, lacunar, or cryptogenic) we recommend treatment with an antiplatelet drug **(Grade 1A)**. Aspirin, the combination of aspirin (25 mg) and extended-release dipyridamole (200 mg twice a

day), and clopidogrel (75 mg daily) are all acceptable options for initial therapy. We recommend an aspirin dose of 50 to 100 mg per day over higher aspirin doses **(Grade 1B)**.

2. In patients who have experienced a non-cardioembolic stroke or TIA, we recommend using the combination of aspirin and extended-release dipyridamole (25/200 mg twice daily) over aspirin **(Grade 1A),** and suggest clopidogrel over aspirin **(Grade 2B)**.

3. In most patients with a non-cardioembolic stroke or TIA, we recommend avoiding long-term use of the combination of aspirin and clopidogrel **(Grade 1B)**. In those with a recent acute myocardial infarction, other acute coronary syndromes, or a recently placed coronary stent, we recommend clopidogrel plus aspirin (75 to 100 mg) **(Grade 1A)**. The optimal duration of dual antiplatelet therapy depends on the specific cardiac indication.

4. For patients who are allergic to aspirin, we recommend clopidogrel **(Grade 1A)**.

Prevention of Non-Cardioembolic Cerebral Ischemic Events: Oral Anticoagulants

1. For patients with non-cardioembolic stroke or TIA, we recommend antiplatelet agents over oral anticoagulation **(Grade 1A)**.

Prevention of Cerebral Ischemic Events in Patients Undergoing Carotid Endarterectomy: Antiplatelet Agents

1. In patients undergoing carotid endarterectomy, we recommend aspirin (50 to 100 mg/d) prior to, and following, the procedure **(Grade 1A)**.

Prevention of Cardioembolic Cerebral Ischemic Events

1. In patients with atrial fibrillation who suffered a recent stroke or TIA, we recommend long-term oral anticoagulation (target INR of 2.5; range: 2.0 to 3.0) **(Grade 1A)**.

2. For patients with cardioembolic stroke who have contraindications to anticoagulant therapy, we recommend aspirin at a dose of 75 to 325 mg/d **(Grade 1B)**.

3. In patients with stroke associated with aortic atherosclerotic lesions, we recommend antiplatelet therapy over no therapy **(Grade 1A)**. For patients with cryptogenic stroke associated with mobile aortic arch thrombi, we suggest either oral anticoagulation or antiplatelet agents **(Grade 2C)**.

4. In patients with cryptogenic ischemic stroke and a PFO, we recommend antiplatelet therapy over no therapy **(Grade 1A)** and suggest antiplatelet agents over anticoagulation **(Grade 2A)**.

5. In patients with mitral valve strands or prolapse, who have a history of TIA or stroke, we recommend antiplatelet therapy **(Grade 1A)**.

Anticoagulation for Cerebral Venous Sinus Thrombosis

1. In patients with venous sinus thrombosis, we recommend that clinicians use UFH **(Grade 1B)** or low-molecular weight heparin **(Grade 1B)** over no anticoagulant therapy during the acute phase, even in the presence of hemorrhagic infarction. In these patients, we recommend continued use of vitamin K antagonist therapy for up to 12 months (target INR: 2.5; range: 2.0 to 3.0) **(Grade 1B)**.

14 CORONARY HEART DISEASE

The discussion of coronary heart disease covers acute treatment of non–ST-segment elevation acute coronary syndromes (ACS) and ST-segment elevation acute coronary artery syndromes, and long-term treatment of post–ST-segment elevation and non–ST-segment elevation ACS. Patients with acute chest pain are identified as having an acute coronary syndrome (ACS) and then differentiated further into those with or without ST-segment elevation. The early treatment decisions are based on this important distinction.

NON–ST-SEGMENT ELEVATION ACUTE CORONARY SYNDROMES

This chapter addresses antithrombotic treatment for patients with non–ST-segment elevation acute coronary syndromes (NSTE ACS), including those undergoing percutaneous coronary intervention (PCI). The diagnoses of NSTE ACS [UA and non–ST-segment elevation myocardial infarction (NSTEMI)] are made retrospectively, after a period of observation.

Patients with NSTE ACS benefit from both antiplatelet and anticoagulant therapy, but in contrast to patients with ST-segment elevation myocardial infarction (MI), they do not benefit from fibrinolytic therapy.

Treatment decisions are influenced by the estimated level of risk of major ischemic events in the days through to the first month following acute presentation.

Classifying Patients According to Risk
Moderate-risk patients will have at least one of:

- ongoing chest pain
- hemodynamic instability
- positive cardiac biomarkers

- dynamic electrocardiogram (ECG) changes

High-risk patients have at least two of the features listed for moderate-risk patients.

Low-risk patients have none of the features listed for moderate-risk patients.

ACUTE MANAGEMENT

Antiplatelet Agents

Aspirin

The Antithrombotic Trialists' Collaboration analysis included 5,031 patients with unstable angina (UA) and reported that aspirin was associated with a 46% relative odds reduction in adverse vascular events. The risk of gastrointestinal bleeding increases with aspirin dose, but its efficacy is equivalent, or even superior, at lower doses.

Thienopyridines

Based on a better safety profile, clopidogrel has essentially replaced ticlopidine. The antiplatelet effect of clopidogrel is delayed after drug administration, but can be achieved more rapidly by giving a loading dose.

The benefit of the combination of clopidogrel and aspirin, particularly among high-risk patients, is now clearly established. In the Clopidogrel in Unstable Angina to Prevent Recurrent Events (CURE) trial, the combination of clopidogrel and aspirin was compared to aspirin alone: the composite outcome of death from cardiovascular causes, non-fatal MI, or stroke was reduced by 20% in the combination group. Major bleeding was significantly more common in clopidogrel-treated patients [relative risk (RR) 1.38; $p = .001$]. Bleeding associated with coronary artery bypass grafting (CABG) was higher among patients receiving clopidogrel within 5 days of surgery (RR 1.53; $p = .06$).

Combination therapy with clopidogrel and aspirin is particularly effective in patients having PCI and stenting.

Dipyridamole

Currently, there is no evidence that dipyridamole is effective in patients with NSTE ACS.

Glycoprotein IIb-IIIa Inhibitors

Three glycoprotein (GP) IIb-IIIa inhibitors are approved for clinical use: abciximab, a monoclonal antibody fragment; eptifibatide, a peptide inhibitor; and tirofiban, a peptidomimetic inhibitor. Abciximab and eptifibatide are indicated as adjunctive antithrombotics in patients undergoing PCI, including those with ACS, while eptifibatide and tirofiban are approved for use at the time of presentation or diagnosis among patients presenting with NSTE ACS.

Abciximab
Abciximab is highly effective in PCI patients. Although major bleeding is increased, the risk is reduced without loss of efficacy by lowering the dose of heparin. Patients presenting with ACS who are not treated with PCI do not appear to benefit from treatment with abciximab. Abciximab does not prevent late restenosis and does not reduce complication rates associated with saphenous venous graft interventions.

Eptifibatide
Although the initial study evaluating eptifibatide in patients undergoing PCI failed to demonstrate efficacy, subsequent studies using higher doses reported that eptifibatide is effective in ACS patients undergoing PCI.

Tirofiban
Two moderate-size trials have reported that tirofiban is effective in NSTE ACS.

Anticoagulant Therapy

Unfractionated Heparin
Unfractionated heparin (UFH) has been evaluated in combination with aspirin in several clinical trials in patients with unstable angina and NSTEMI. A pooled analysis showed that, compared with aspirin, the combination of heparin and aspirin resulted in a relative risk of 0.44 for death/MI.

Low-Molecular-Weight Heparin
In placebo-controlled randomized trials, the low-molecular-weight heparin (LMWH) preparations nadroparin and dalteparin were shown to be effective in the short term in NSTE ACS.

Of the LMWH preparations tested, enoxaparin has been evaluated most extensively in NSTE ACS. A systematic overview of six randomized trials compared the relative efficacy and bleeding of enoxaparin and UFH in 21,946 patients with NSTE ACS. There was no difference in death at 30 days (3.0% versus 3.0%) but there was a significant reduction in the 30-day composite of death or MI favoring enoxaparin over UFH (10.1% versus 11.0%; odds ratio: 0.91). There were no significant differences in major bleeding.

More recently, the Superior Yield of the New Strategy of Enoxaparin, Revascularization and Glycoprotein IIb/IIIa Inhibitors (SYNERGY) trial compared enoxaparin and UFH in 10,027 high-risk NSTE ACS patients intended to receive an early invasive strategy. There were no differences in ischemic events between the treatment groups, but major bleeding was significantly increased with enoxaparin.

Low-Molecular-Weight Heparin and Percutaneous Coronary Intervention

In several small studies, enoxaparin appeared to be safe when used in combination with tirofiban or eptifibatide during PCI. Favorable outcomes have also been reported with the combination of dalteparin and abciximab in patients undergoing PCI.

Fondaparinux

The indirect factor Xa inhibitor fondaparinux has been evaluated in a large phase III study in patients with NSTE ACS.

In the Fifth Organization to Assess Strategies in Acute Ischemic Syndromes (OASIS-5) trial, a randomized, blinded, double-dummy trial, fondaparinux was compared with enoxaparin in 20,078 patients with NSTE ACS. During PCI, there was an algorithm to supplement anticoagulation in both study arms with additional UFH. The primary outcome measure, the composite of death, MI, or refractory ischemia at nine days, was similar in both groups (5.8% for fondaparinux versus 5.7% for enoxaparin). There was significantly less major bleeding with fondaparinux than enoxaparin (2.2% versus 4.1%, $p < .001$). At 180 days, there were fewer deaths (5.8% versus 6.5%; hazard ratio: 0.89) and a reduction in the death or MI composite (10.5% versus 11.4%; HR: 0.92) in the fondaparinux arm. Although there was an increased risk of coronary guide-catheter thrombus formation with fondaparinux compared with enoxaparin (0.9% versus 0.4%; $p = .001$) the rates of death or MI were similar between the groups in this population. A strategy of providing additional UFH boluses as per the local standard (for example 50 to 60 IU/kg UFH) during PCI has been reported to decrease the risk of catheter thrombosis.

Direct Thrombin Inhibitors

A systematic overview of seven randomized trials including 30,154 patients compared direct thrombin inhibitors with UFH in patients with NSTE ACS or undergoing PCI. Treatment with a direct thrombin inhibitor was associated with a reduction in death or MI, compared with UFH (3.7% vs 4.6%; OR: 0.80). Similar reductions were observed in PCI trials (3.0% vs 3.8%; OR: 0.79).

The risk reduction in death or MI at the end of treatment was similar in trials comparing hirudin or bivalirudin with UFH, but there was a slight excess of events with univalent thrombin inhibitors. When major bleeding outcomes were analyzed by agent, hirudin was associated with an excess of major bleeding compared with UFH, whereas both bivalirudin and univalent thrombin inhibitors were associated with lower rates of major bleeding.

RECOMMENDATIONS

Antiplatelet Therapies

1. For all patients presenting with NSTE ACS, without a clear allergy to aspirin, we recommend immediate aspirin (162 to 325 mg orally) and then daily oral aspirin (75 to 100 mg) **(Grade 1A)**.
2. For all NSTE ACS patients with an aspirin allergy, we recommend immediate treatment with clopidogrel, 300 mg oral bolus, followed by 75 mg daily, indefinitely **(Grade 1A)**.
3. For NSTE ACS patients who are at moderate or greater risk (eg, ongoing chest pain, hemodynamic instability, positive troponin, or dynamic ECG changes) for an ischemic event and who will undergo an early invasive management strategy (ie, diagnostic catheterization followed by anatomy-driven revascularization):
   a. We recommend "upstream" treatment, either with clopidogrel (300 mg oral bolus, followed by 75 mg daily) or a small-molecule intravenous (IV) GP IIb-IIIa inhibitor (eptifibatide or tirofiban) **(Grade 1A)**.
   b. We suggest "upstream" use of both clopidogrel and a small-molecule IV GP IIb-IIIa inhibitor **(Grade 2A)**. Scrupulous attention to weight- and renal-based dosing algorithms must be part of eptifibatide or tirofiban administration.
   c. For patients presenting with NSTE ACS, we recommend against abciximab as initial treatment except when coronary anatomy is known and PCI is planned within 24 hours **(Grade 1A)**.
4. For NSTE ACS patients who are at moderate or greater risk for an ischemic event and for whom an early conservative or a delayed invasive strategy of management is to be used:
   a. We recommend "upstream" treatment with clopidogrel (300 mg oral bolus, followed by 75 mg daily) **(Grade 1A)**.
   b. We suggest "upstream" use of both clopidogrel and a small-molecule IV GP IIb-IIIa inhibitor **(Grade 2B)**.
5. For NSTE ACS patients who undergo PCI, we recommend treatment with both clopidogrel and an IV GP IIb-IIIa inhibitor **(Grade 1A)**.

a. We recommend a loading dose of 600 mg of clopidogrel given at least 2 hours prior to planned PCI followed by 75 mg daily **(Grade 1B)**.

b. If ticlopidine is given, we suggest that a loading dose of 500 mg be given at least 6 hours before planned PCI **(Grade 2C)**.

c. For PCI patients who cannot tolerate aspirin, we suggest that the loading dose of clopidogrel (600 mg) or ticlopidine (500 mg) be given at least 24 hours prior to planned PCI **(Grade 2C)**.

d. We recommend use of a GP IIb-IIIa antagonist (abciximab or eptifibatide) **(Grade 1A)** for all NSTE ACS patients with at least moderate risk features undergoing PCI in whom a GP IIb-IIIa inhibitor has not been started "upstream." We recommend administration of abciximab as a 0.25 mg/kg bolus followed by a 12-hour infusion at a rate of 10 μg/min **(Grade 1A)** and eptifibatide as a double bolus (each 180 μg/kg, given 10 minutes apart) followed by an 18-hour infusion of 2.0 μg/kg/min **(Grade 1A)**. Appropriate dose reduction of eptifibatide must be based upon renal function.

e. In patients undergoing PCI in whom a GP IIb-IIIa inhibitor has not been started upstream, we recommend against the use of tirofiban as an alternative to abciximab **(Grade 1B)**.

6. For NSTE ACS patients who have received clopidogrel and are scheduled for coronary bypass surgery, we suggest discontinuing clopidogrel for at least 5 days prior to the scheduled surgery **(Grade 2A)**.

Anticoagulant Therapies

1. For all patients presenting with NSTE ACS, we recommend anticoagulation with UFH or LMWH or bivalirudin or fondaparinux over no anticoagulation **(Grade 1A)**.

a. We recommend weight-based dosing of UFH and maintenance of the activated partial thromboplastin time (APTT) between 50 and 70 seconds **(Grade 1B)**.

b. We recommend against routine monitoring of the anticoagulant effect of LMWH **(Grade 1C)**. Careful attention is needed to appropriately adjust LMWH dose in patients with renal insufficiency.

2. For NSTE ACS patients who will undergo an early invasive strategy of management (ie, diagnostic catheterization followed by anatomy-driven revascularization):

a. We recommend UFH (with a GP IIb-IIIa inhibitor) over either LMWH or fondaparinux **(Grade 1B)**.

b. We suggest bivalirudin over UFH in combination with a thienopyridine as an initial antithrombotic strategy in patients with moderate- to high-risk features presenting with a NSTE ACS and scheduled for very early coronary angiography (less than 6 hours) **(Grade 2B)**.

3. For NSTE ACS patients in whom an early conservative or a delayed invasive strategy of management is to be used:

   a. We recommend fondaparinux over enoxaparin **(Grade 1A)**. For patients treated with "upstream" fondaparinux and undergoing PCI, we recommend that additional IV boluses of UFH be given at the time of the procedure (for example, 50 to 60 U/kg) as well as additional IV doses of fondaparinux (2.5 mg if also receiving a GP IIb-IIIa inhibitor, and 5 mg, if not) **(Grade 1B)**. Additionally, PCI operators should regularly flush the catheters with UFH during the procedure as well.

   b. We recommend LMWH over UFH **(Grade 1B)**. We recommend continuing LMWH during PCI treatment of patients with NSTE ACS when LMWH has been started as the "upstream" anticoagulant **(Grade 1B)**. If the last dose of enoxaparin was given ≤ 8 hours prior to PCI, we recommend no additional anticoagulant therapy **(Grade 1B)**. If the last dose of enoxaparin was given 8 to 12 hours before PCI, we recommend a 0.3 mg/kg bolus of IV enoxaparin at the time of PCI **(Grade 1B)**.

4. In low- to moderate-risk patients with NSTE ACS undergoing PCI, we recommend either bivalirudin with provisional ("bail-out") GP IIb-IIIa inhibitors or UFH plus a GP IIb-IIIa inhibitor over alternative antithrombotic regimens **(Grade 1B)**.

ACUTE ST-SEGMENT ELEVATION MYOCARDIAL INFARCTION

Acute ST-segment elevation myocardial infarction (STEMI) is usually caused by an occluded epicardial infarct-related artery (IRA). Reperfusion therapy is highly effective and can be achieved either with fibrinolysis or percutaneous coronary intervention. Antiplatelet and antithrombotic therapy are also effective in patients with an acute coronary syndrome.

Reperfusion Therapy

Reperfusion with primary percutaneous coronary intervention can be achieved in 80 to 95% of cases. PCI is more effective than fibrinolysis.

In an overview of 20 randomized trials comparing PCI with fibrinolytic therapy in patients with STEMI, patients assigned to PCI had lower short-term mortality rates (5% vs 7%; OR: 0.70, $p = .038$), nonfatal MI (3% vs 6%; OR; 0.42) and ICH (0.05% vs 1.0%; OR: 0.05, $p < .0001$). There was an increased risk for major bleeding in patients undergoing primary percutaneous coronary intervention (PCI) (7% vs 5%; OR: 1.3, $p = .032$). These short-term benefits of primary PCI over fibrinolytic therapy appear to be sustained.

Despite the proven benefits of primary PCI, fibrinolytic therapy will continue to have a pivotal role in reperfusion therapy because timely access to optimal primary PCI is limited.

Fibrinolysis

Fibrinolytic therapy benefits patients with STEMI who are treated within 12 hours of symptom onset. There is no evidence that fibrinolytic therapy is of benefit for patients with normal ECG or non-specific changes, and there is some suggestion of harm for patients with ST-segment depression only.

The overview from Fibrinolytic Therapy Trialists' (FTT) analysis of fibrinolysis versus control ($n = 58,600$) reported 18 fewer deaths per 1,000 patients treated. Benefit was observed among patients presenting with ST-segment elevation or bundle-branch block (BBB)—irrespective of age, sex, blood pressure (if less than 180 mm Hg systolic), or a previous history of myocardial infarction or diabetes. The benefit of fibrinolysis is substantially higher in patients presenting within 2 hours after symptom onset than in those presenting later. To take advantage of this observation, studies were performed evaluating prehospital fibrinolysis, an approach made more feasible by the availability of bolus therapy with either reteplase or tenecteplase.

A meta-analysis of six trials comparing prehospital-initiated fibrinolysis with conventional in-hospital strategy ($n = 6,434$) found that the prehospital-initiated group received earlier treatment (mean 104 vs 162 minutes; $p = .007$) and had a significant reduction in all-cause hospital mortality (OR: 0.83, $p = .03$).

Hemorrhage is the most important risk of fibrinolytic therapy, especially intracranial hemorrhage, which is fatal in up to two-thirds of patients. The risk of ICH is reduced by lowering the dosage of adjunctive IV heparin.

Comparison of Fibrinolytic Agents

All four fibrinolytic agents [streptokinase, tissue plasminogen activator (t-PA), reteplase, and tenecteplase] have been evaluated in large clinical trials and are effective. Streptokinase and t-PA are given by continuous IV infusion, whereas reteplase and tenecteplase are given as bolus injection, thereby providing the latter two with a convenience advantage. Alteplase (t-PA), was shown to be more effective than streptokinase in the Global Utilization of Streptokinase and Tissue Plasminogen Activator for Occluded Coronary Arteries (GUSTO) trial. In two separate trials, reteplase showed similar efficacy and safety as streptokinase and t-PA. Tenecteplase showed similar efficacy and similar safety to t-PA, although tenecteplase appeared to cause less ICH than t-PA in high-risk patients.

Antiplatelet/Antithrombotic Therapy

In order to maintain IRA patency, adjunctive antiplatelet and antithrombotic treatments should be included in the management of acute STEMI, regardless of the reperfusion strategy initially employed.

Aspirin

Aspirin is very effective and safe in patients with ACS. Treatment should be initiated as early as possible—at the time of initial contact with health care personnel. In the Second International Study of Infarct Survival (ISIS-2) trial, 162.5 mg of aspirin daily reduced five-week vascular mortality (9.4% vs 11.8%; OR: 23%, $p < .00001$). When aspirin was combined with streptokinase, the mortality benefit was significantly better than either agent alone.

A meta-analysis of 14 other trials ($n = 19,288$) demonstrated a significant reduction (about 30%) in serious vascular events and in total mortality in patients assigned antiplatelet (mainly aspirin), compared to control.

Clopidogrel

Two large trials demonstrated that clopidogrel added to aspirin (and other standard therapy) is effective in acute STEMI. Clopidogrel as Adjunctive Reperfusion Therapy (CLARITY), a double-blind randomized trial, enrolled 3,491 patients within 12 hours of symptom onset. Patients received aspirin, fibrinolysis, and, for those receiving fibrin-specific lytic agents, heparin and either clopidogrel of placebo. Treatment with clopidogrel resulted in a significant (36%) reduction in the odds of an occluded infarct-related artery on the angiogram (at 2 to 8 days), or early death or recurrent myocardial infarction. By 30 days, treatment with clopidogrel reduced the risk of cardiovascular death, recurrent myocardial infarction, or recurrent ischemia leading to urgent revascularization by 20% ($p = .03$). The incidence of major bleeding was low in both treatment arms (1.3% in the clopidogrel group vs 1.1% in the placebo group).

The ClOpidogrel and Metoprolol in Myocardial Infarction Trial (COMMIT) performed in China evaluated clopidogrel in addition to 162 mg of aspirin daily in 45,852 patients with suspected MI. About 50% received fibrinolysis, and 75% received an anticoagulant. Treatment with clopidogrel resulted in a 9% relative risk reduction ($p = .002$) in the incidence of death, reinfarction, or stroke at a follow-up of approximately 2 weeks. There was no difference between the two groups in fatal bleeding, blood transfused, or ICH.

Anticoagulants

Unfractionated Heparin
The benefits of UFH in STEMI are very modest when added to aspirin. In an overview analysis of seven trials comparing the combination of aspirin and heparin [subcutaneous (SC) or IV] with aspirin alone (93% of patients also received fibrinolytic therapy), the patients assigned to heparin had 5 (±2) fewer deaths (p = .03), 3 (±1) fewer reinfarctions (p = .04), and 1 (±0.4) fewer pulmonary emboli (p = .01), 1 (±1) more strokes, and 3 (±1) more major bleeds (p < .001) per 1,000 patients treated.

Six randomized, controlled trials have compared IV UFH with no heparin in STEMI treated with fibrinolysis (n = 1,735). In-hospital mortality was similar (5.1% vs 5.6%; OR: 0.91), as were rates of recurrent ischemia and reinfarction. The risk of total bleeding was significantly higher in the UFH group (22.7% vs 16.2%; OR: 1.55). There was no significant difference in the effects of heparin among patients receiving t-PA, streptokinase, or anistreplase, or between patients who did and did not receive aspirin.

Despite the limited evidence for its efficacy, it is standard practice to use IV UFH as adjunctive therapy in STEMI patients. The optimal dosing regimens and duration of treatment are uncertain.

Low-Molecular-Weight Heparin
LMWH has been compared to placebo or to UFH in the setting of fibrinolysis in several randomized trials.

Pooled analysis of four small studies (n = 1,376) comparing LMWH to placebo found no difference in mortality, but showed an increase in major bleeding (3.6% vs 1.0%; OR: 3.00)

The Clinical Trial of Metabolic Modulation in Acute Myocardial Infarction Treatment Evaluation (CREATE) study, a randomized, double-blind, placebo-controlled trial of over 15,000 patients presenting within 12 hours of symptom onset, compared LMWH (reviparin) to placebo for 7 days. Aspirin was used in 97% of patients, clopidogrel or ticlopidine in 55%, fibrinolytic therapy in 73%. The seven-day composite endpoint of death, myocardial reinfarction, or stroke was reduced in the reviparin group (9.6% vs 11.0%; HR: 0.87, p = .005). There were also significant reductions in mortality (8.0% vs 8.9%; HR: 0.89, p = .04) and reinfarction (1.6% vs 2.1%; HR: 0.75 p = .02). There was a small, significant excess of hemorrhagic strokes in the reviparin group (0.3% vs 0.1%, p = .03). At 30 days, both composite outcomes were similarly reduced, including death, reinfarction, or disabling stroke. There was a significant increase in the rates of life-threatening or major bleeding at 7 days with reviparin, which was accounted for mainly by those patients undergoing reperfusion therapy.

In a pooled analysis of five trials ($n = 7,960$) that compared enoxaparin to UFH as an adjunct to fibrinolysis, there was no difference in mortality (5.8% vs 6.1%), but there was a reduction in reinfarction (3.2% vs 5.1%; OR: 0.61; 95% CI: 0.48 to 0.76) and an increase in major bleeds (3.2% vs 2.3%; OR: 1.38; 95% CI: 1.05 to 1.81) in the enoxaparin group.

The Enoxaparin and Thrombolysis Reperfusion for Acute Myocardial Infarction Treatment, Thrombolysis in Myocardial Infarction-Study 25 (ExTRACT-TIMI 25) trial was a double-blind, double-dummy comparison of enoxaparin ($n = 10,256$) administered for a median of 7 days with UFH ($n = 10,223$) for a median of 2 days. The primary endpoint (30-day composite of all-cause mortality and nonfatal reinfarction) was significantly lower in the enoxaparin group (9.9% vs 12%; RR: 0.83, $p <$ .001). The benefit of enoxaparin was evident at 48 hours. The benefit with enoxaparin was offset by a significant increase in 30-day major and minor bleeding.

Fondaparinux

Fondaparinux has been evaluated in the Sixth Organization to Assess Strategies in Acute Ischemic Syndrome (OASIS-6) study. This large ($n = 12,092$) randomized double-blind trial compared fondaparinux and control for up to 8 days in patients with STEMI. Randomization was stratified by indication for the use or non-use of UFH. Stratum 1 (5,658 patients) did not receive UFH and stratum 2 (6,434 patients) received UFH. The composite of death or MI was significantly reduced at 9 days (7.4% vs 8.9%; HR: 0.83, $p =$ .003), at 30 days (primary outcome; 9.7% vs 11.2%; HR: 0.86, $p =$ .008), and at study end (3 to 6 months) (10.5% vs 11.5%; HR: 0.88, $p =$ .008) in the fondaparinux compared to the control group. Within stratum 1, patients receiving fondaparinux had a significantly lower death or reinfarction rate when compared with placebo. In stratum 2 (those with an indication for UFH), there was no difference between fondaparinux and UFH. This lack of effect was caused by an increase in death or reinfarction among patients who underwent primary PCI ($n = 3,768$). In contrast, those patients in stratum 2 who did not undergo primary PCI ($n = 2,666$), showed a trend towards benefit with fondaparinux as compared to unfractionated heparin (eg, at day 30: 11.5% vs 13.8%; HR: 0.82, $p =$ .08).

Among patients who did not receive any initial reperfusion therapy, fondaparinux was superior to control (placebo or UFH) in reducing 30-day death or reinfarction (12.2% vs 15.1%, $p <$ .05). Similarly, among patients who received fibrinolytic therapy ($n = 5,436$), fondaparinux was significantly better than control (placebo or UFH; 10.9% vs 13.6%,

$p < .05$). There was a non-significant trend toward fewer severe bleeds with fondaparinux compared with the control group (placebo or UFH). The rates of ICH were similar in the two groups (0.2% vs 0.2%).

In patients undergoing primary PCI, in the patients assigned to fondaparinux, there was a higher rate of guiding catheter thrombosis (0 vs 22, $p < .001$) and more coronary complications (abrupt coronary artery closure, new angiographic thrombus, catheter thrombus, no reflow, dissection, or perforation (225 vs 270, $p = .04$). These differences were not as striking among patients who received UFH prior to primary PCI ($n = 496$; catheter thrombus in 2 patients receiving fondaparinux compared to no patients receiving UFH). In the 231 fondaparinux patients who underwent a PCI (other than primary) in hospital (for whom UFH was recommended prior to the procedure), there were no catheter-related thrombi seen.

Direct Thrombin Inhibitors

Direct thrombin inhibitors have been evaluated in acute coronary syndromes, including STEMI patients receiving fibrinolysis. A meta-analysis that included individual patient data ($n = 9,947$) from five trials found significant reduction in the endpoint of recurrent MI with direct thrombin inhibitors, compared with IV UFH (2.5% vs 3.4%; OR: 0.75). This reduction was seen with hirudin and bivalirudin and not with univalent agents. Overall mortality, however, was similar with adjunctive direct thrombin inhibitor, as was the combined endpoint of death and recurrent MI.

In addition to the studies in the meta-analysis, the Hirulog and Early Reperfusion or Occlusion (HERO-2) trial compared IV bivalirudin and IV UFH for at least 48 hours post-streptokinase in STEMI patients ($n = 17,073$). Bivalirudin did not reduce the primary 30-day mortality endpoint (10.8% vs 10.9%; OR: 0.99) but reduced the rate of reinfarction at 96 hours (1.6% vs 2.3%; OR: 0.70, $p = .001$). Rates of major bleeding (1.4% vs 1.1%; OR: 1.32, $p = .05$) and minor bleeding (12.8% vs 9.0%; OR: 1.47 $p < .0001$) were significantly higher with bivalirudin.

Glycoprotein IIb-IIIa Inhibitors

In STEMI patients, results of clinical trials do not support the use of GP IIb-IIIa inhibitors as the sole means of reperfusion (ie, without fibrinolysis or in conjunction with primary PCI).

The GUSTO V trial randomized STEMI patients ($n = 16,588$) within 6 hours of symptom onset to receive a standard dose of abciximab, or a combination of abciximab for 12 hours with half-dose of reteplase. The primary end point of 30-day mortality was similar in both groups. Bleeding was significantly higher with combination therapy.

A meta-analysis of three trials (including GUSTO V; $n = 23,166$) found no difference in 30-day or 6- to 12-month mortality between those receiving abciximab and half-dose fibrinolysis compared to those receiving full-dose fibrinolysis. Major bleeding rates were significantly higher in patients receiving abciximab.

GP IIb-IIIa receptor inhibitors have been studied as adjunctive antiplatelet therapy in STEMI patients undergoing PCI. A meta-analysis of eight randomized trials ($n = 3,949$) found that abciximab was associated with a significant reduction in 30-day (2.4% vs 3.4%; OR: 0.68, $p = .047$) and 6- to 12-month mortality (4.4% vs 6.2%; OR: 0.69, $p = .01$). The rates of bleeding were similar in both groups.

FACILITATED PCI

Facilitated PCI refers to a strategy of planned, immediate PCI after an initial pharmacologic regimen such as half- or full-dose fibrinolysis, a GP IIb-IIIa inhibitor, or a combination of reduced-dose fibrinolysis plus a GP IIb-IIIa inhibitor.

Six randomized trials, including two double-blinded, placebo-controlled studies, were included as part of a quantitative review in which primary PCI ($n = 1,487$) was compared with facilitated PCI ($n = 1,466$).

The overall mortality was significantly increased in the facilitated, compared with the primary, PCI group (5.6% vs 4.0%; OR: 1.43, $p = .042$). Reinfarction and short-term target vessel revascularization were also significantly higher in the facilitated group.

Combination Reduced-Dose Fibrinolysis and GP IIb-IIIa Inhibitors

Half-dose fibrinolysis (reteplase or tenecteplase) combined with a standard dose of GP IIb-IIIa inhibitor has been compared with standard doses of GP IIb-IIIa inhibitor prior to primary PCI. The primary endpoint in one trial (infarct size) was not reduced with the facilitated combination compared with abciximab alone, and there was no difference in mortality, reinfarction, or urgent target vessel revascularization.

RESCUE PCI

Rescue (also known as salvage) PCI is defined as PCI within 12 hours after failed fibrinolysis for patients with continuing or recurrent myocardial ischemia. A meta-analysis has been performed of five randomized trials comparing PCI to a conservative approach after failed fibrinolysis in patients ($n = 920$) with STEMI.

Mortality tended to be lower with rescue PCI compared to conservative therapy (6.9% vs 10.7%; OR; 0.63, p = .055) within the first 30 days of follow-up. There was also a reduction of the combined endpoint of death or reinfarction in favor of rescue PCI at both short-term and longer-term follow-up. Rescue PCI was associated with substantially and significantly more major bleeding (11.9% vs 1.3%, OR 9.05, p<0.001).

RECOMMENDATIONS

Reperfusion Therapy

1. For patients with ischemic symptoms characteristic of acute myocardial infarction of ≤ 12 hours duration and persistent ST elevation, we recommend that all undergo rapid evaluation for reperfusion (primary PCI or fibrinolytic) therapy and have a reperfusion strategy implemented promptly after contact with the health-care system **(Grade 1A)**.

Fibrinolysis

1. In patients with acute MI who are candidates for fibrinolytic therapy, we recommend administration as soon as possible (ideally within 30 minutes) after arrival to the hospital or first contact with the health-care system **(Grade 1A)**.

2. In health-care settings where prehospital administration of fibrinolytic therapy is feasible, we recommend prehospital administration of fibrinolytic therapy **(Grade 1A)**.

3. For patients with ischemic symptoms characteristic of acute myocardial infarction of ≤ 12 hours duration, and persistent ST elevation, we recommend administration of streptokinase, anistreplase, alteplase, reteplase, or tenecteplase over no fibrinolytic therapy **(all Grade 1A)**.

4. For patients with symptom duration ≤ 6 hours, we recommend the administration of alteplase **(Grade 1A)** or tenecteplase **(Grade 1A)**, and suggest reteplase **(Grade 2B)** over streptokinase.

5. For patients receiving fibrinolytic therapy, we suggest the use of a bolus agent (eg, tenecteplase) to facilitate the ease of administration and potentially reduce the risk of nonintracranial hemorrhage-related bleeding (tenecteplase, **Grade 2A**).

6. For patients with ischemic symptoms characteristic of acute myocardial infarction of ≤ 12 hours duration, a left bundle branch block (LBBB) with associated ST segment changes, we recommend fibrinolytic therapy if primary PCI is not readily available **(Grade 1B)**.

7. For patients with ischemic symptoms characteristic of acute myocardial infarction of ≤ 12 hours duration and ECG findings consistent with a

true posterior MI, we suggest fibrinolytic therapy if primary PCI is not readily available **(Grade 2B)**.

8. For high-risk patients with ongoing symptoms characteristic of acute myocardial infarction or hemodynamic compromise and duration of 12 to 24 hours who have persistent ST elevation or LBBB with ST segment changes, we suggest fibrinolytic therapy if primary PCI is not readily available **(Grade 2B)**.

9. In patients with any history of ICH, or with a history of head trauma, or with ischemic stroke within the past 6 months, we recommend *against* administration of fibrinolytic therapy **(Grade 1C)**.

Antiplatelet/Antithrombotic Therapy

Aspirin

1. For patients with acute ST-elevation MI, whether or not they receive fibrinolytic therapy, we recommend aspirin (160 to 325 mg orally) over no aspirin therapy at initial evaluation by health-care personnel **(Grade 1A)** followed by indefinite therapy (75 mg to 162 mg orally daily) **(Grade 1A)**.

Clopidogrel

1. For patients with acute STEMI, we recommend clopidogrel in addition to aspirin **(Grade 1A)**. The recommended dosing for clopidogrel is 300 mg orally for patients age ≤ 75 years and 75 mg orally for patients age > 75 years if they receive fibrinolytic agents or no reperfusion therapy, followed by 75 mg orally daily for up to 28 days **(Grade 1A)**.

2. For patients with acute STEMI who have not received a coronary stent, we suggest that clopidogrel 75 mg daily could be continued beyond 28 days and up to 1 year **(Grade 2B)**.

3. For patients undergoing primary PCI, we suggest clopidogrel in addition to aspirin, with a recommended initial dosing of at least 300 mg **(Grade 1B)**, followed by 75 mg daily (for the duration of therapy).

Antithrombin Therapy

1. For patients with acute STEMI, in addition to aspirin and other antiplatelet therapies, we recommend the use of antithrombin therapy over no antithrombin therapy **(Grade 1A)**, including for those patients receiving fibrinolysis (and regardless of which lytic agent is administered), primary PCI, or patients not receiving reperfusion therapy.

Unfractionated Heparin

1. For patients receiving streptokinase, we suggest administration of either IV UFH (5,000 U bolus followed by 1,000 U/h for patients > 80 kg, 800 U/h for < 80 kg) with a target APTT of 50 to 75 seconds or subcutaneous UFH (12,500 U every 12 hours) over no UFH therapy for 48 hours **(both Grade 1B)**.

2. For patients receiving alteplase, tenecteplase, or reteplase for fibrinolysis in acute myocardial infarction, we recommend administration of weight-adjusted heparin [60 U/kg bolus for a maximum of 4,000 U, followed by 12 U/kg/h (1,000 U/h maximum)] adjusted to maintain an APTT of 50 to 70 seconds for 48 hours **(Grade 1B)**.

3. For patients with STEMI undergoing primary PCI, we recommend administration of IV UFH over no UFH therapy **(Grade 1C)**. The recommended periprocedural dosing in patients receiving a GP IIb-IIIa inhibitor is 50 to 70 U/kg [target activated clotting time (ACT) > 200 seconds]; in patients not receiving a GP IIb-IIIa inhibitor, the recommended periprocedural dosing is 60 to 100 U/kg (target ACT 250 to 350 seconds).

Low-Molecular-Weight Heparin

1. For patients with acute STEMI, regardless of whether or not they receive reperfusion therapy, we recommend the use of reviparin over no therapy **(Grade 1B)**. Recommended dosing for reviparin is 3,436 IU for < 50 kg, 5,153 IU for 50 to 75 kg, or 6,871 IU for > 75 kg every 12 hours SC for up to 7 days. For patients undergoing primary PCI, UFH should be used periprocedurally and reviparin initiated 1 hour post-sheath removal.

2. For patients with acute STEMI receiving fibrinolytic therapy who have preserved renal function [> 2.5 mg/dL (220 μmol/L) in males and < 2.0 md/dL (175 μmol/L) in females], we recommend the use of enoxaparin over unfractionated heparin, continued up to 8 days **(Grade 2A)**. Recommended dosing for enoxaparin is for age < 75 years, 30 mg IV bolus followed by 1 mg/kg SC every 12 hours (maximum 100 mg for the first two SC doses); and for age ≥ 75 years, no IV bolus, 0.75 mg/kg SC every 12 hours (maximum 75 mg for the first two SC doses).

Fondaparinux

1. For patients with acute STEMI who are not receiving reperfusion therapy, we recommend fondaparinux over no therapy **(Grade 1A)**. Recommended dosing for fondaparinux is 2.5 mg IV for the first dose and then SC once daily for up to 9 days.

2. For patients with acute STEMI receiving fibrinolytic therapy and thought not to have an indication for anticoagulation, we recommend fondaparinux over no therapy (2.5 mg IV for the first dose and then SC once daily up to 9 days) **(Grade 1B)**.
3. For patients with acute STEMI receiving fibrinolytic therapy and thought to have an indication for anticoagulation, we suggest fondaparinux (2.5 mg IV for the first dose and then SC once daily for up to 9 days) could be used as an alternative to UFH **(Grade 2B)**.
4. For patients with acute ST-elevation MI and undergoing primary PCI, we recommend *against* using fondaparinux **(Grade 1A)**.

Direct Thrombin Inhibitors
1. For patients with acute STEMI treated with streptokinase, we suggest clinicians *not* use bivalirudin as an alternative to unfractionated heparin **(Grade 2B)**.

Glycoprotein IIb-IIIa Inhibitors
1. For patients with acute STEMI, we recommend *against* the combination of standard-dose abciximab and half-dose reteplase or tenecteplase with low-dose IV UFH over standard-dose reteplase or tenecteplase **(Grade 1B)**.
2. For patients with acute STEMI, we suggest clinicians *not* use the combination of streptokinase and any GP IIb-IIIa inhibitor **(Grade 2B)**.
3. For patients with acute STEMI undergoing primary PCI (with or without stenting), we recommend the use of abciximab **(Grade 1B)**. Recommended dosing for abciximab is 0.25 mg/kg IV bolus followed by 0.125 µg/kg/min (maximum 10 µg/min) for 12 hours.

Facilitated PCI
1. For patients with acute STEMI undergoing primary PCI, we recommend *against* the use of fibrinolysis, with or without a GP IIb-IIIa inhibitor **(Grade 1B)**.
2. For patients with acute STEMI who are to undergo primary PCI, we suggest administration of a GP IIb-IIIa inhibitor prior to coronary angiography **(Grade 2B)**. The largest number of patients studied in this setting received abciximab 0.25 mg/kg IV bolus followed by 0.125 µg/kg/min (maximum 10 µg/min) for 12 hours; recommended dosing for eptifibatide is two 180 µg IV boluses (10 minutes apart) followed by 2.0 µg/kg/min infusion for 12 to 24 hours; recommended dosing for tirofiban is 25 µg/kg IV bolus followed by 0.15 µg/kg/min for 24 hours.

Rescue PCI

1. For patients with STEMI who have received fibrinolysis but who have persistent STE (< 50% resolution 90 minutes after treatment initiation compared with the pretreatment ECG), we recommend rescue PCI should be performed over repeat fibrinolysis or no additional reperfusion therapy **(Grade 1B)**, and suggest it be done as soon as possible and within 2 hours of identification of lack of STE resolution **(Grade 2C)**.

15 PRIMARY AND SECONDARY PREVENTION OF CHRONIC CORONARY ARTERY DISEASE

This chapter considers the treatment of the following patient groups: (1) post–ST-segment elevation acute coronary syndrome (ACS); (2) Post–non–ST-segment elevation ACS; (3) post-percutaneous coronary intervention (PCI); (4) stable coronary artery disease (CAD); (5) congestive heart failure; and (6) persons with coronary heart disease (CHD) risk factors.

POST–ST-SEGMENT ELEVATION AND NON–ST-ELEVATION TREATMENT

Antiplatelet Therapy

Short-term Antiplatelet Therapy Trials

ISIS-2 showed that, in myocardial infarction (MI) patients treated with fibrinolytic therapy, the short-term reduction in reinfarction persisted for at least a mean of 15 months. Aspirin reduced the risk of nonfatal reinfarction by 49% and nonfatal stroke by 46%.

The Clopidogrel as Adjunctive Reperfusion Therapy (CLARITY), Thrombolysis in Myocardial Infarction 28 (TIMI 28), and Clopidogrel and Metoprolol in Myocardial Infarction (COMMIT) trials evaluated the addition of clopidogrel to antithrombotic therapy with aspirin, heparin, and a fibrinolytic agent. In the CLARITY trial, the addition of a loading dose of 300 mg of clopidogrel followed by 75 mg/d was associated with a significant 36% reduction in the composite primary endpoint of death, MI, or an occluded infarct-related coronary artery ($p < .001$) at the time of angiography. The Chinese COMMIT trial of 45,852 patients with acute MI, half of whom received reperfusion therapy, demonstrated benefit from clopidogrel 75 mg/d compared with placebo; both groups received aspirin. The primary endpoint of death, MI, or stroke was reduced by 9% ($p = .002$) and mortality was reduced by 7% ($p = .03$).

Long-Term Antiplatelet Therapy Trials

The Antiplatelet Trialists' (APT) Collaboration update included 18,788 patients with a history of MI. Allocation to antiplatelet therapy for a mean duration of 27 months resulted in a 25% odds reduction ($p < 0$) in serious vascular events. The overall benefits were larger than the excess risk of major extracerebral hemorrhage. These data also provided support for administration of an aspirin dose of 75 to 100 mg daily for cardiovascular disease treatment.

Aspirin and Clopidogrel for Secondary Prevention

The Clopidogrel for High Atherothrombotic Risk and Ischemic Stabilization, Management, and Avoidance (CHARISMA) trial compared the efficacy and safety of clopidogrel plus aspirin against aspirin alone in patients at high risk for a cardiovascular event. In the total population of 15,603 patients, there was a non-significant trend toward benefit from combined antiplatelet therapy.

Long-term Anticoagulant Therapy

A systematic overview of anticoagulation therapy with a vitamin K antagonist (VKA) in patients with coronary artery disease showed that moderate-intensity and high-intensity anticoagulation therapy was effective in reducing the incidence of MI and stroke, compared with control subjects, but at a cost of increased bleeding. Although in three early trials aspirin appeared to be at least as effective as and safer than VKA therapy, recent evidence indicates that aspirin is less effective than VKA. In these recent trials, both high-intensity warfarin (INR: 3.0 to 4.0) and moderate-intensity warfarin (INR: 2.0 to 2.5) plus aspirin (80 mg/d) was better than aspirin (80 mg/d) alone. In contrast, a combination of low or moderate fixed-dose warfarin and aspirin was found to be no more effective, but to cause more bleeding than aspirin. Thus, both high-intensity (INR: 3.0 to 4.0) warfarin and moderate-intensity warfarin plus aspirin is more effective but causes more bleeding than aspirin alone for long-term treatment of MI patients.

Antiplatelet Therapy After PCI

Dual antiplatelet therapy reduces the rate of ischemic events after PCI, and dual antiplatelet therapy is indicated for an extended duration until the high early risk of stent thrombosis diminishes. Thereafter, PCI patients should be treated with aspirin indefinitely. Although the risk of major bleeding with dual antiplatelet therapy is increased, the benefit of combination therapy outweighs the risk.

Triple Antithrombotic Therapy

Treatment of patients with coronary stents is problematic when they also require treatment with VKA [eg, because of associated atrial fibrillation (AF), mechanical heart valve replacement, or other indications for long-term VKA therapy]. The therapeutic dilemma is based on the following observations: stent thrombosis is more likely when clopidogrel is withheld; it is likely that stroke risk (in AF and mechanical valve patients) increases if VKA is withdrawn after stenting; and there is an increased risk of bleeding when VKAs are added to aspirin or clopidogrel, or to both. Consideration should be given to the placement of a bare metal stent to minimize the duration of triple therapy.

Heart Failure

Patients with heart failure are at increased risk of venous thromboembolism and of systemic embolism. There is no convincing evidence, however, that patients with heart failure of non-ischemic cause and who are in sinus rhythm benefit from antithrombotic therapy.

ANTITHROMBOTIC THERAPY IN PREVENTION OF GRAFT OCCLUSION

Saphenous Vein Grafts

Off-pump versus On-pump Coronary Artery Bypass Graft

A meta-analysis of five randomized trials comparing off-pump coronary artery bypass (OPCAB) versus on-pump coronary bypass surgery reported a modest reduction in graft patency with OPCAB procedures (odds ratio: 1.51; $p = .003$).

Treatment with Antiplatelet Agents: Aspirin

A systematic review by the Antiplatelet Trialists' Collaboration found that aspirin, especially when initiated early, was associated with improved graft patency for an average of 1 year after surgery. Two randomized trials have shown that the combination of clopidogrel and aspirin is more effective than aspirin alone in patients who undergo coronary artery bypass surgery. In contrast, there appears to be no benefit from the combination of aspirin and dipyridamole over aspirin alone on graft patency.

Aprotinin in Coronary Bypass Surgery

The antifibrinolytic agent aprotinin has been reported to reduce postoperative bleeding after bypass surgery. The safety of this drug in bypass surgery has been questioned based on publication of an observational study involving 4,374 patients who underwent surgical revascularization. Aprotinin use was associated with an increase in postoperative renal failure, in MI and ischemic stroke, and five-year mortality. Neither aminocaproic acid nor tranexamic acid use was associated with an increased mortality.

Internal Mammary Bypass Grafts

The data for prevention of internal mammary artery (IMA) bypass graft occlusion following coronary artery bypass graft (CABG) is limited to subgroup analysis of relatively small studies investigating bypass grafting with both venous and arterial grafts. Although the results are inconclusive, aspirin is indicated because of its efficacy in patients with coronary artery disease.

PRIMARY PREVENTION OF CARDIOVASCULAR EVENTS

Aspirin

Five large trials have investigated acetylsalicylic acid (ASA, or aspirin) in subjects (mainly men) free of a history of previous major vascular events (MI or stroke), and one trial investigated this question in women. Aspirin therapy reduced ischemic cardiac events in four of the five trials, the effect being most marked for nonfatal MI and among patients with a cardiac profile that placed them at a greater than 10% risk of an event in a 10-year period. A meta-analysis reported that aspirin was associated with a relative risk reduction (RRR) in all cardiovascular events of 15%, an RRR in MI of 30%, and a non-significant RRR of 6% in all-cause mortality. Aspirin increased the relative risk of stroke by 6% (not significant), and increased the relative risk of bleeding complications significantly—by 69%. The results of the analysis suggest that aspirin is safe and worthwhile for primary prevention in subjects who are at a risk of 1.5% per annum for a major coronary episode; safe, but of limited value, at a coronary event risk of 1.0% per annum; and unsafe at a risk of 0.5%.

Primary Prevention in Women

Women have a lower baseline risk of ischemic events than men. In the Women's Health Study (WHS) there was a non-significant reduction of 9% ($p = .13$) in cardiovascular events, and a 17% reduction in the risk of stroke in the aspirin group, compared with the placebo group ($p = .04$). Gastrointestinal bleeding requiring transfusion increased in the aspirin group [risk reduction 1.40 ($p = .02$)]. In subgroup analyses, there were significant reductions in major cardiovascular events, ischemic stroke, and myocardial infarction among women who were 65 years or over (in whom the risk of the primary endpoint was reduced by 26% due to aspirin). There was a greater benefit from aspirin among former smokers and those who had never smoked than in current smokers. Women aged 45 to 54 years did not benefit from routine aspirin administration for primary prevention.

A sex-specific meta-analysis of randomized controlled trials that included a total of 51,342 women reported that aspirin therapy was associated with a significant 12% reduction in cardiovascular events ($p = .03$) and a 17% reduction in stroke ($p = .02$).

Dual Antiplatelet Therapy

In CHARISMA, dual antiplatelet therapy (with clopidogrel and aspirin) was less effective than aspirin alone in the subgroup of patients with multiple risk factors.

Vitamin K Antagonists

The results of the Thrombosis Prevention Trial indicate that low-intensity warfarin (targeted INR: 1.5) has similar efficacy to ASA for the prevention of all ischemic heart disease (IHD) outcomes, and that warfarin is particularly effective in reducing fatal events. A combination of warfarin and aspirin was even more effective in reducing ischemic cardiac events, but at the price of an increase in hemorrhagic stroke. Compared with placebo, the risk of non-cerebral major bleeding was increased to a similar degree by aspirin, warfarin, and a combination of the two.

RECOMMENDATIONS

1. For patients with acute coronary syndromes with and without ST-segment elevation, we recommend ASA given initially at a dose of 75 to 162 mg and then indefinitely at a dose of 75 to 100 mg daily **(Grade 1A)**.

2. For patients with ST-segment elevation ACS, with or without fibrinolytic therapy, we recommend clopidogrel, administered as a 300 mg oral loading dose for patients ≤ 75 years of age, a 75 mg starting dose for those > 75 years of age, and continued at a daily dose of 75 mg for 2 to 4 weeks **(Grade 1A)**. We suggest continuing clopidogrel for up to 12 months following hospital discharge **(Grade 2B)**.

3. For patients with non–ST elevation ACS, we recommend combination therapy with aspirin (75 to 100 mg daily) and clopidogrel (75 mg daily) for 12 months **(Grade 1A)**.

4. For patients in whom ASA is contraindicated or not tolerated, we recommend clopidogrel monotherapy for long-term administration (75 mg daily) **(Grade 1A)**.

5. For patients with symptomatic coronary artery disease, we suggest aspirin (75 to 100 mg daily) in combination with clopidogrel (75 mg daily) **(Grade 2B)**.
6. For most patients (all except the high-risk group described in recommendations below) in most health-care settings, following ACS, we recommend ASA alone (75 to 100 mg daily) over oral Vitamin K antagonists alone or in combination with aspirin **(Grade 1B)**.
7. For most patients after MI, in health-care settings in which meticulous INR-monitoring and highly skilled VKA dose titration are expected and widely accessible, we suggest long-term (up to 4 years) high-intensity oral VKA (target INR: 3.5, range: 3.0 to 4.0) without concomitant aspirin or moderate intensity oral VKA (target INR: 2.5, range: 2.0 to 3.0) with aspirin ($\le$ 100 mg/d) over aspirin alone **(both Grade 2B)**.
8. For high-risk patients with myocardial infarction, including those with a large anterior MI, those with significant heart failure, those with intra-cardiac thrombus visible on transthoracic echocardiography, those with atrial fibrillation, and those with a history of a thromboembolic event, we suggest the combined use of moderate-intensity (INR: 2.0 to 3.0) oral VKA plus low-dose aspirin ($\le$ 100 mg daily) for at least 3 months after the MI **(Grade 2A)**.
9. For long-term treatment of patients after PCI, we recommend aspirin at a dose of 75 to 100 mg daily **(Grade 1A)**.
10. For patients undergoing PCI with bare metal stents (BMS) placement, we recommend aspirin (75 to 100 mg daily) plus clopidogrel over aspirin alone **(Grade 1A)**.
11. For patients undergoing PCI with BMS placement following ACS, we recommend 12 months of aspirin (75 to 100 mg daily) plus clopidogrel (75 mg daily) over aspirin alone **(Grade 1A)**.
12. For patients undergoing PCI with drug eluting stents (DES), we recommend aspirin (75 to 100 mg daily) plus clopidogrel (75 mg daily for at least 12 months (**Grade 1A** for 3 to 4 months; **Grade 1B** for 4 to 12 months). Beyond 1 year, we suggest continued treatment with aspirin plus clopidogrel indefinitely, if there are no bleeding or other tolerability issues **(Grade 2C)**.
13. For patients undergoing stent placement with a strong concomitant indication for VKA, we suggest triple antithrombotic therapy **(Grade 2C)**. We suggest 4 weeks of clopidogrel following BMS, and 1 year following DES **(Grade 2C)**.
14. For recommendations for the use of antiplatelet agents in other patient populations with atrial fibrillation, see Chapter 11 (Antithrombotic Therapy in Atrial Fibrillation).

15. For patients after stent placement, we suggest clopidogrel **(Grade 1A)** or ticlopidine **(Grade 2B)** over cilostazol. We recommend clopidogrel over ticlopidine **(Grade 1A)**.

16. For aspirin-intolerant patients undergoing PCI, we recommend use of a thienopyridine derivative rather than dipyridamole **(Grade 1B)**.

17. For patients who undergo PCI with no other indication for VKA, we recommend against VKA **(Grade 1A)**.

18. In patients with congestive heart failure due to a non-ischemic etiology, we recommend against routine use of aspirin or oral VKA **(Grade 1B)**.

19. For all patients with coronary artery disease undergoing CABG, we recommend aspirin, 75 to 100 mg/d, indefinitely **(Grade 1A)**. We suggest that the aspirin be started postoperatively **(Grade 2A)**.

20. For patients undergoing CABG, we recommend against addition of dipyridamole to aspirin therapy **(Grade 1A)**.

21. For patients with coronary artery disease undergoing CABG who are allergic to aspirin, we recommend clopidogrel, 300 mg, as a loading dose 6 hours after the operation, followed by 75 mg/d orally, indefinitely **(Grade 1B)**.

22. In patients who undergo CABG following non–ST-segment elevation ACS, we suggest clopidogrel, 75 mg/d, for 9 to 12 months following the procedure, in addition to treatment with aspirin **(Grade 2B)**.

23. For patients who have received clopidogrel for ACS and are scheduled for coronary bypass surgery, we suggest discontinuing clopidogrel for 5 days prior to the scheduled surgery **(Grade 2A)**.

24. For patients undergoing CABG who have no other indication for VKA, we recommend clinicians not administer VKA **(Grade 1C)**.

25. For patients undergoing CABG in whom oral anticoagulants are indicated, such as those with heart valve replacement, we suggest clinicians administer VKA in addition to aspirin **(Grade 2C)**.

26. For all patients with coronary artery disease who undergo IMA bypass grafting, we recommend aspirin, 75 to 162 mg/d, indefinitely **(Grade 1A)**.

27. For all patients undergoing IMA bypass grafting who have no other indication for VKAs, we recommend against using VKAs **(Grade 1C)**.

28. For patients with at least moderate risk for a coronary event (based on age and cardiac risk factor profile with a 10-year risk of a cardiac event of > 10%), we recommend 75 to 100 mg aspirin daily over either no antithrombotic therapy or VKA **(Grade 2A)**.

29. For patients at particularly high risk of events, in whom INR can be monitored without difficulty, we suggest low-dose VKA (target INR: approximately 1.5) over aspirin therapy **(Grade 2A)**.

30. For all patients, we recommend against the routine addition of clopidogrel to aspirin therapy in primary prevention **(Grade 1A)**. For patients with an aspirin allergy who are at moderate to high risk for a cardiovascular event, we recommend monotherapy with clopidogrel **(Grade 1B)**.
31. For women < 65 years of age who are at risk for an ischemic stroke and in whom the concomitant risk of major bleeding is low, we suggest aspirin at a dose of 75 to 100 mg daily over no aspirin therapy **(Grade 2A)**.
32. For women > 65 years of age at risk for ischemic stroke or MI and in whom the concomitant risk of major bleeding is low, we suggest aspirin at a dose of 75 to 100 mg daily over no aspirin therapy **(Grade 2B)**.

Patients (particularly those in the highest risk groups) for whom systems permitting meticulous monitoring of anticoagulant therapy are available, who place a relatively high value on small absolute risk reductions in coronary events, and who are not influenced by an element of inconvenience and potential bleeding risk associated with VKA, are likely to derive the greatest overall benefit from administration of VKA rather than aspirin.

16 ANTITHROMBOTIC THERAPY IN PERIPHERAL ARTERIAL OCCLUSIVE DISEASE

Atherosclerotic peripheral arterial disease (PAD) is often asymptomatic. If symptomatic, it usually presents as intermittent claudication, less commonly as rest pain, and uncommonly as limb gangrene. The prevalence of PAD increases with age, occurring in 2 to 3% of men and 1 to 2% of women over the age of 60 years. Most patients with intermittent claudication remain unchanged or improved, but 20 to 30% progress, and less than 3% eventually require amputation. Chronic renal insufficiency, diabetes mellitus, and heavy smoking are risk factors for progression of PAD.

PAD patients have a two- to threefold increased risk of cardiovascular and stroke mortality. Mortality and morbidity in PAD can be reduced by controlling key risk factors such as smoking, dyslipidemia, and hypertension.

ANTIPLATELET THERAPY

Antithrombotic therapy lowers the incidence of stroke and myocardial infarction and may modify the natural history of PAD, but does not appear to delay progression of atherosclerosis.

Aspirin

The Antithrombotic Trialists' Collaboration meta-analysis of 42 trials found that, among 9,214 patients with PAD, there was a 23% reduction in serious vascular events ($p = .004$) in patients treated with antiplatelet therapy (mainly aspirin). The Physicians Health Study, a primary prevention study, found that aspirin 325 mg every other day decreased the need for peripheral arterial reconstructive surgery, but it did not influence the development of intermittent claudication.

Ticlopidine

Ticlopidine reduces the risk of fatal and nonfatal cardiovascular events in patients with intermittent claudication.

Clopidogrel

Clopidogrel was more effective than aspirin in the Clopidogrel vs Aspirin in Patients at Risk of Ischemic Events (CAPRIE) trial in patients with symptomatic PAD than in those enrolled with cardiac or cerebrovascular disease, but the interpretation of this subgroup analysis is controversial.

Picotamide

A thromboxane A2 synthase inhibitor and thromboxane A2 receptor blocker, picotamide has been compared with placebo and with aspirin in separate randomized trials. Picotamide was more effective than placebo in reducing major and minor cardiovascular events and in preventing progression of carotid atherosclerosis (as measured by B-mode ultrasonography). In patients with type II diabetes with PAD, picotamide was more effective than aspirin in reducing two-year mortality (3.0% vs 5.5%). The incidence of bleeding was no different between picotamide and aspirin, although gastrointestinal side effects were more common with aspirin. Picotamide is approved for use in some European countries.

ANTICOAGULANT THERAPY

A Cochrane review of three studies [two evaluating vitamin K antagonist (VKA), one evaluating unfractionated heparin (UFH)] reported no significant effect on overall mortality or cardiovascular events. Anticoagulants did not improve symptoms of intermittent claudication. Major and minor bleeding events were significantly more frequent in patients treated with VKA compared to control, with a non-significant increase in fatal bleeding.

OTHER TREATMENTS

Patients with intermittent claudication show improvement with exercise treatment.

The vasodilator cilostazol, a type III phosphodiesterase inhibitor, increases maximal walking distance and pain-free walking distance. Cilostazol is more effective in increasing walking distance than pentoxifylline.

Pentoxifylline, a drug that increases red blood cell deformity and decreases whole-blood viscosity, has been reported to improve pain-free walking distance, but the results of studies have not been consistent.

Early reports of benefit from prostaglandins in patients with critical limb ischemia have not been borne out in more recent randomized trials.

ACUTE LIMB ISCHEMIA

Acute arterial occlusion can be either embolic or thrombotic. Most emboli arise from the heart, and prompt embolectomy is very effective. Thrombotic occlusions are usually associated with advanced atherosclerosis. Since the affected limbs often have a well-developed collateral blood supply, an acute occlusion can be silent and, even when it is symptomatic, the presentation is less dramatic than that caused by embolic occlusion.

Anticoagulants
It is standard practice to treat patients with thromboembolic arterial occlusion and acute limb ischemia with heparin, although the benefits of heparin have never been demonstrated in a formal clinical trial.

Thrombolysis
Systemic thrombolysis has been replaced by catheter-directed thrombolysis. The results of randomized trials comparing catheter-directed thrombolysis to surgical intervention showed similar mortality and amputation rates in both groups. Thrombolysis was found to reduce the need for open major surgical procedures, but caused more bleeding and was associated with a higher rate of distal embolization.

There is no convincing evidence that any one thrombolytic agent is better or safer than another.

LOWER EXTREMITY RECONSTRUCTION

Prosthetic grafts for large-caliber arteries, such as the aorta, iliac, and femoral vessels, have excellent long-term patency and durability. Adjunctive antithrombotic therapy is generally not necessary to maintain patency. In contrast, smaller-caliber infrainguinal bypasses (femoral-popliteal/tibial) have a diminished long-term patency. Autogenous venous conduits are preferable over prosthetic grafts for these infrainguinal bypasses.

Both venous and prosthetic grafts are at risk for early occlusion from technical problems and for intermediate and late occlusions from neointimal hyperplasia and progression of atherosclerosis in the native vascular beds.

Perioperative dextran does not improve the long-term patency of bypass grafts, and results of studies with extended postoperative treatment with LMWH or with VKA are inconclusive.

There is evidence that antiplatelet therapy extends the patency of peripheral bypass grafts. A meta-analysis of 11 studies, demonstrated a significant risk reduction of graft occlusion of 32% in patients who were given platelet inhibitors. Furthermore, a meta-analysis of five trials comparing aspirin (alone or combined with other antiplatelet therapy) with placebo in infrainguinal bypass surgery found a 22% risk reduction in occlusion.

Infrainguinal Autogenous Vein Bypasses

A multicenter, randomized trial reported that saphenous vein grafts have a better patency rate at 4 years than expanded polytetrafluoroethylene (PTFE) prostheses (49% vs 12%).

A Cochrane systematic review of the effects of antiplatelet therapy on patency of peripheral grafts concluded that aspirin had a slight beneficial effect overall, but the benefit was weaker for vein grafts. Ticlopidine has been reported to improve patency of femoropopliteal and femorotibial bypasses, but clopidogrel has not been evaluated for this indication. Although not conclusive, there is some evidence that antiplatelet therapy should be started preoperatively. Results of studies on the value of VKA, used alone or in combination with aspirin, are inconclusive.

Infrainguinal Prosthetic Grafts

Antiplatelet therapy appears to be more effective for maintaining patency of prosthetic grafts than of vein grafts. The limited evidence suggests VKAs are less effective and cause more bleeding than aspirin.

CAROTID ENDARTERECTOMY

Studies with indium-111-labeled platelets indicate that platelets accumulate at the endarterectomy site immediately after operation. The intensity of platelet accumulation decreases over time. In a randomized, double-blind trial, aspirin started preoperatively was associated with a marked reduction in intra- and postoperative stroke.

ASYMPTOMATIC CAROTID STENOSIS

There is indirect evidence that aspirin might be beneficial in patients with advanced stenosis who do not undergo carotid endarterectomy. However, there is no evidence that dual antiplatelet therapy is effective for this indication.

LOWER EXTREMITY PROCEDURES

The evidence that antiplatelet therapy prolongs patency of peripheral arterial endovascular procedures is inconclusive and there is no evidence that anticoagulants are effective in prolonging patency.

RECOMMENDATIONS

Chronic Limb Ischemia and Intermittent Claudication

1. In PAD patients with clinically manifest coronary or cerebrovascular disease, we recommend lifelong antiplatelet therapy over no antiplatelet therapy **(Grade 1A)**.
2. In those without clinically manifested coronary or cerebrovascular disease, we suggest aspirin (75 to 100 mg daily) over clopidogrel **(Grade 2B)**. In patients who are aspirin-intolerant, we recommend clopidogrel over ticlopidine **(Grade 1B)**.
3. In patients with PAD and intermittent claudication, we recommend against the use of anticoagulants to prevent vascular mortality or cardiovascular events **(Grade 1A)**.
4. For patients with moderate to severe, disabling intermittent claudication, who do not respond to exercise therapy and who are not candidates for surgical or catheter-based intervention, we recommend cilostazol **(Grade 1A)**. We suggest that clinicians not use cilostazol in those with less disabling claudication **(Grade 2A)**. We recommend against the use of pentoxifylline **(Grade 2B)**.
5. For patients with intermittent claudication, we recommend against the use of anticoagulants **(Grade 1A)**.
6. For patients with limb ischemia, we suggest clinicians do not use prostaglandins **(Grade 2B)**.
7. In patients who suffer from acute arterial emboli or thrombosis, we recommend immediate systemic anticoagulation with UFH over no anticoagulation **(Grade 1C)**. In patients undergoing embolectomy, we

suggest systemic anticoagulation with UFH followed by long-term anticoagulation with VKA **(Grade 2C)**.

8. In patients with short-term (< 14 days) thrombotic or embolic disease, we suggest intra-arterial thrombolytic therapy **(Grade 2B)**, provided patients are at low risk of myonecrosis and ischemic nerve damage developing during the time needed to achieve revascularization by this method.

9. For patients undergoing major vascular reconstructive procedures, we recommend intravenous UFH, prior to the application of vascular cross clamps **(Grade 1A)**.

10. For all patients undergoing infrainguinal arterial reconstruction, we recommend aspirin (75 to 100 mg, begun preoperatively) **(Grade 1A)**. We recommend against the routine use of perioperative dextran, heparin, or long-term anticoagulation with VKA for all extremity reconstructions **(Grade 1B)**.

11. For patients receiving routine autogenous vein infrainguinal bypass, we recommend aspirin (75 to 100 mg, begun preoperatively) **(Grade 1A)**. We suggest that VKA not be used routinely in patients undergoing infrainguinal vein bypass **(Grade 2B)**. For those at high risk of bypass occlusion and limb loss, we suggest VKA plus aspirin **(Grade 2B)**.

12. For patients receiving routine *prosthetic* infrainguinal bypass, we recommend aspirin (75 to 100 mg, begun preoperatively) **(Grade 1A)**. We suggest that VKA not be used routinely in patients undergoing prosthetic infrainguinal bypass **(Grade 2A)**.

13. In patients undergoing carotid endarterectomy, we recommend that aspirin, 75 to 100 mg, be given preoperatively to prevent perioperative ischemic neurologic events. We recommend lifelong postoperative aspirin (75 to 100 mg daily) **(Grade 1A)**.

14. In nonoperative patients with asymptomatic carotid stenosis (primary or recurrent), we recommend lifelong aspirin, 75 to 100 mg mg/d **(Grade 1C)**. In this patient group, we recommend against dual antiplatelet therapy with aspirin and clopidogrel **(Grade 1B)**.

15. For patients undergoing lower-extremity balloon angioplasty (with or without stenting), we recommend long-term aspirin (75 to 100 mg/d) **(Grade 1C)**. For patients undergoing lower-extremity balloon angioplasty (with or without stenting), we recommend against anticoagulation with heparin or VKA **(Grade 1A)**.

17 VENOUS THROMBOEMBOLISM, THROMBOPHILIA, AND PREGNANCY

Anticoagulant therapy is indicated during pregnancy for the prevention and treatment of VTE, for the prevention and treatment of systemic embolism in patients with mechanical heart valves, and, in combination with aspirin, for the prevention of recurrent pregnancy loss in women with antiphospholipid antibodies. The use of anticoagulant therapy during pregnancy is challenging because of the potential for fetal, as well as maternal, complications.

Since the last review, there is new information on the following: the risk of VTE in pregnant women with thrombophilia, the management of pregnant women with prior VTE, the treatment of VTE in pregnancy, the safety of low-molecular-weight heparin (LMWH) during pregnancy, the difficulties of managing pregnant women with mechanical heart valves, the relationship between thrombophilia and pregnancy complications, and the value of anticoagulant therapy in this setting.

VITAMIN K ANTAGONISTS

Vitamin K antagonists cross the placenta and have the potential to cause fetal wastage, bleeding in the fetus, and teratogenicity. Estimates of the incidence of warfarin-induced congenital fetal anomalies vary widely, but the true incidence is likely to be low. The typical defect is nasal hypoplasia and stippled epiphyses, with limb hypoplasia occurring less commonly. Embryopathy typically occurs after in utero exposure to vitamin K antagonists during the first trimester of pregnancy, particularly between the 6th and 12th week. The substitution of heparin at, or prior to, 6 weeks appears to eliminate the risk of embryopathy.

Exposure to vitamin K antagonists during any trimester has also been associated with central nervous system abnormalities, but these complications are likely to be rare. Minor neurodevelopmental problems have also been described in children exposed to coumarins in the second and third trimester of pregnancy, but their significance is uncertain. Warfarin-mediated fetal coagulopathy can cause bleeding in the neonate at the time of delivery. This complication can be minimized or avoided by substituting warfarin with heparin or LMWH 2 weeks before delivery. Warfarin does not pass into breast milk and can be taken by women who require postpartum anticoagulant therapy.

Unfractionated heparin (UFH) or LMWH may not provide adequate protection against thrombosis in pregnant patients with prosthetic heart valves, and, under certain circumstances, the use of warfarin may be considered. If warfarin is considered during pregnancy, the patient should be informed about the potential risks and of the statement made in the package insert by the manufacturers that warfarin is contraindicated during pregnancy.

Women being treated with long-term warfarin and who are planning to become pregnant can be managed either by performing frequent pregnancy tests and substitution of warfarin with UFH or LMWH when pregnancy is diagnosed or by replacing the warfarin with UFH or LMWH before conception is attempted.

UNFRACTIONATED HEPARIN AND LOW-MOLECULAR-WEIGHT HEPARIN

Neither UFH nor LMWH crosses the placenta and they are therefore safe for the fetus and should be used as necessary for maternal indications. Long-term use of heparin can be complicated by osteopenia and, uncommonly, by symptomatic osteoporosis. This complication occurs less frequently with LMWH.

Adjusted-dose heparin has been reported to provide inadequate protection in patients with mechanical prosthetic heart valves, as has weight-adjusted LMWH. It is uncertain whether the reported failures with heparin or LMWH were caused by inadequate dosing or an inherent limitation of these anticoagulants in pregnant women with prosthetic heart valve patients. If heparin is used in patients with high-risk prosthetic heart valves, it should be administered in high doses with careful laboratory monitoring. If LMWH is used, it should be given in therapeutic, weight-adjusted doses, administered twice daily to achieve anti-factor Xa levels of 1.0 to 1.2 U/mL 4 to 6 hours after subcutaneous injection.

OTHER PARENTERAL ANTICOAGULANTS

The available literature suggests that danaparoid is safe during pregnancy, but the quality of evidence available to support that claim is low. The safety of r-hirudin and of pentasaccharide in pregnancy is uncertain.

ASPIRIN

Although animal studies have shown that aspirin may increase the risk of congenital anomalies, clinical data suggest that low-dose aspirin during the second and third trimester is safe for the fetus and, although less certain, is likely to be safe in the first trimester. There might be a small increase in the risk of neonatal bleeding if aspirin is used close to term in doses of 325 mg or more per day. The combination of aspirin and either UFH or LMWH is effective in reducing pregnancy loss in women with antiphospholipid antibodies and a history of recurrent or late pregnancy loss. In patients at high risk of pre-eclampsia, aspirin is also effective in reducing that risk.

RECOMMENDATIONS

Vitamin K Antagonist Exposure In Utero

1. For women receiving anticoagulation for the management of VTE who become pregnant, we recommend that vitamin K antagonists be substituted with UFH or LMWH **(Grade 1A)**.

2. For women with mechanical valves who become pregnant, we suggest either adjusted-dose LMWH or UFH twice daily throughout pregnancy or adjusted-dose LMWH or UFH twice daily until the 13th week, with substitution by vitamin K antagonists until LMWH or UFH are resumed close to delivery **(Grade 1C)**. In pregnant women with high-risk mechanical valves (eg, older generation valve in the mitral position or history of thromboembolism), we suggest the use of oral anticoagulants over heparin **(Grade 2C)**.

Management of Women Receiving Long-Term Vitamin K Antagonists Who Are Considering Pregnancy

1. For women requiring long-term vitamin K antagonists who are attempting pregnancy and who are candidates for UFH or LMWH substitution, we suggest performing frequent pregnancy tests and substituting UFH or LMWH for vitamin K antagonists when pregnancy is achieved **(Grade 2C)**.

Anticoagulant Exposure During Breast-Feeding

1. For lactating women using warfarin or UFH who wish to breast-feed, we recommend continuing these medications **(Grade 1A)**.

2. For lactating women using LMWH, danaparoid, or r-hirudin who wish to breast-feed, we suggest continuing these medications **(Grade 2C)**.

3. For breast-feeding women, we suggest alternative anticoagulants rather than pentasaccharides **(Grade 2C)**.

LMWH Therapy

1. For pregnant patients, we suggest LMWH over UFH for the prevention and treatment of VTE **(Grade 2C)**.

Risk of Venous Thromboembolism Following Cesarean Section

1. We suggest that a thrombosis risk assessment be carried out in all women undergoing cesarean section to determine the need for thromboprophylaxis **(Grade 2C)**.

2. In patients without additional thrombosis risk factors undergoing cesarean section, we recommend against the use of specific thromboprophylaxis other than early mobilization **(Grade 1B)**.

Thromboprophylaxis Following Cesarean Section

1. For women considered at increased risk of VTE after cesarean section because of the presence of at least one risk factor in addition to pregnancy and cesarean section, we suggest pharmacologic thromboprophylaxis (prophylactic LMWH or UFH) or mechanical prophylaxis (graduated compression stockings or intermittent pneumatic compression) while in hospital following delivery **(Grade 2C)**.

2. For women with multiple additional risk factors for thromboembolism who are undergoing cesarean section and considered to be at very high risk of VTE, we suggest that pharmacologic prophylaxis be combined with the use of graduated compression stockings and/or intermittent pneumatic compression **(Grade 2C)**.

3. For selected high-risk patients in whom significant risk factors persist following delivery, we suggest extended prophylaxis (up to 4 to 6 weeks post-delivery) following discharge from hospital **(Grade 2C)**.

Treatment of Venous Thromboembolism During Pregnancy

1. For pregnant women with acute VTE, we recommend initial therapy with either adjusted-dose subcutaneous LMWH or adjusted-dose UFH [intravenous bolus, followed by a continuous infusion to maintain the activated partial thromboplastin time (APTT) within the therapeutic range or subcutaneous therapy adjusted to maintain the APTT 6 hours postinjection into the therapeutic APTT range] for at least 5 days **(Grade 1A)**.

2. For pregnant women with acute VTE, after initial therapy, we recommend that subcutaneous LMWH or UFH be continued throughout pregnancy **(Grade 1B)**.

3. For pregnant women with acute VTE, we suggest that anticoagulants be continued for at least 6 weeks postpartum (for a minimum total duration of 6 months) **(Grade 2C)**.

4. For pregnant women receiving adjusted-dose LMWH or UFH therapy, we recommend discontinuation of the heparin at least 24 hours prior to elective induction of labor **(Grade 1C)**.

Prevention of Recurrent VTE in Pregnant Women

1. For pregnant women with a single episode of VTE associated with a transient risk factor that is no longer present and no thrombophilia, we recommend clinical surveillance antepartum and anticoagulant prophylaxis postpartum **(Grade 1C)**.

2. If the transient risk factor associated with a previous VTE event is pregnancy or estrogen-related, we suggest antepartum clinical surveillance or prophylaxis (prophylactic LMWH/UFH or intermediate-dose LMWH/UFH) plus postpartum prophylaxis, rather than routine care **(Grade 2C)**.

3. For pregnant women with a single idiopathic episode of VTE but without thrombophilia and who are not on long-term anticoagulants, we recommend one of the following rather than routine care or adjusted-dose anticoagulation: prophylactic LMWH/UFH or intermediate-dose LMWH/UFH or clinical surveillance throughout pregnancy plus post-partum anticoagulants **(Grade 1C)**.

4. For pregnant women with thrombophilia (confirmed laboratory abnormality) who have had a single prior episode of VTE and who are not receiving long-term anticoagulants, we recommend one of the following rather than routine care or adjusted-dose anticoagulation: antepartum prophylactic or intermediate-dose LMWH; or prophylactic or intermediate-dose UFH; or clinical surveillance throughout pregnancy plus postpartum anticoagulants **(Grade 1C)**.

5. For women with "higher risk" thrombophilias (eg, antithrombin deficiency, persistent positivity for the presence of antiphospholipid antibodies; compound heterozygosity for prothrombin G20210A variant and factor V Leiden or homozygosity for these conditions) who have had a single prior episode of VTE and who are not receiving long-term anticoagulants, we suggest, in addition to postpartum prophylaxis, antepartum prophylactic or intermediate-dose LMWH, or prophylactic or intermediate-dose UFH, rather than clinical surveillance **(Grade 2C)**.

6. For pregnant women with multiple (≥ 2) episodes of VTE who are not receiving long-term anticoagulants, we suggest antepartum prophylactic, intermediate-dose, or adjusted-dose LMWH, or prophylactic, intermediate, or adjusted-dose UFH followed by postpartum anticoagulants, rather than clinical surveillance **(Grade 2C)**.

7. For pregnant women receiving long-term anticoagulants for prior VTE, we recommend LMWH or UFH throughout pregnancy (either adjusted-dose LMWH or UFH, 75% of adjusted-dose LMWH, or intermediate-dose LMWH) followed by resumption of long-term anticoagulants postpartum **(Grade 1C)**.

8. For all pregnant women with previous DVT, we suggest the use of graduated elastic compression stockings, both ante- and postpartum **(Grade 2C)**.

Risk of Pregnancy-Related VTE in Women With Thrombophilia

1. For pregnant patients with thrombophilia but no prior VTE, we recommend that physicians do not use routine pharmacologic antepartum prophylaxis, but instead, perform an individualized risk assessment **(Grade 1C)**.

Prevention of Pregnancy-Related VTE in Women With Thrombophilia

1. For pregnant women with no prior history of VTE but antithrombin deficiency, we suggest antepartum and postpartum prophylaxis **(Grade 2C)**.
2. For all other pregnant women with thrombophilia and no prior VTE, we suggest antepartum clinical surveillance or prophylactic LMWH or UFH, plus postpartum anticoagulants **(Grade 2C)**.

Risk of Pregnancy Complications in Women With Thrombophilia

1. For women with recurrent early pregnancy loss (three or more miscarriages) or unexplained late pregnancy loss, we recommend screening for antiphospholipid antibodies (APLAs) **(Grade 1A)**.
2. For women with severe or recurrent pre-eclampsia or intrauterine growth retardation (IUGR), we suggest screening for APLAs **(Grade 2C)**.

Prevention of Pregnancy Complications in Women With Thrombophilia

1. For women with APLAs and recurrent (≥ 3) pregnancy loss or late pregnancy loss and no history of venous or arterial thrombosis, we recommend antepartum administration of prophylactic or intermediate-dose UFH or prophylactic LMWH combined with aspirin **(Grade 1B)**.

Prevention of Recurrent Pre-eclampsia in Women With No Thrombophilia

1. For women considered at high risk for pre-eclampsia, we recommend low-dose aspirin therapy throughout pregnancy **(Grade 1B)**.
2. For women with a past history of pre-eclampsia, we suggest that UFH and LMWH not be used as prophylaxis in subsequent pregnancies **(Grade 2C)**.

Anticoagulant Management of Mechanical Prosthetic Valves in Pregnant Women

1. For pregnant women with mechanical heart valves, we recommend that the decision about anticoagulant management during pregnancy include an assessment of additional risk factors for thromboembolism, including valve type, position, and prior history of thromboembolism, and that the decision be strongly influenced by patient preferences **(Grade 1C)**.

2. For pregnant women with mechanical heart valves, we recommend one of the following anticoagulant regimens in preference to no anticoagulation:

   (a) adjusted-dose LMWH twice daily throughout pregnancy **(Grade 1C)**. We suggest that doses be adjusted to achieve the manufacturer's peak anti-factor Xa LMWH 4 hours post–subcutaneous-injection **(Grade 2C)** OR

   (b) adjusted-dose UFH throughout pregnancy administered subcutaneously every 12 hours in doses adjusted to keep the mid-interval APTT at least twice control or attain an anti-factor Xa heparin level of 0.35 to 0.70 U/mL **(Grade 1C)** OR

   (c) UFH or LMWH (as above) until the 13th week, with warfarin substitution until close to delivery, when UFH or LMWH is resumed **(Grade 1C)**.

3. In women judged to be at very high risk of thromboembolism in whom concerns exist about the efficacy and safety of UFH or LMWH as dosed above (eg, older generation prosthesis in the mitral position, or history of thromboembolism), we suggest vitamin K antagonists throughout pregnancy, with replacement by UFH or LMWH (as above) close to delivery, rather than one of the regimens above, after a thorough discussion of the potential risks and benefits of this approach **(Grade 2C)**.

   Remark: For all the recommendations above, usual long-term anticoagulants should be resumed postpartum.

4. For pregnant women with prosthetic valves at high risk of thromboembolism, we recommend the addition of low-dose aspirin, 75 to 100 mg/d **(Grade 2C)**.

18 ANTITHROMBOTIC THERAPY IN NEONATES AND CHILDREN

Compared to the adult population, thromboembolism (TE) is uncommon in children, but in when it occurs, it can be devastating. Adequately powered clinical trials in the prevention and treatment of TE in children are sparse and difficult to perform. Accordingly, most recommendations for antithrombotic therapy in pediatrics have been extrapolated from results of clinical trials performed in adults, and should not be considered definitive. The dosing and choice of antithrombotic agents in children are influenced by many factors specific to the pediatric population. These pediatric-specific factors include differences in the pharmacokinetics and pharmacodynamics of drugs, difficulties in compliance, difficulties in venous access, and difficulties in obtaining pediatric formulations of a number of agents.

CATHETER AND VENOUS LINE THROMBOSIS

Over 80% of venous thromboembolic events [VTEs] are secondary to central venous lines (CVL). These lines, which are placed either into the umbilical veins or upper arm veins, lead to complicating thrombosis in over 10% of neonates. The effectiveness of anticoagulants in preventing acute or chronic complications of CVL–thrombosis has not been evaluated.

SYSTEMIC VENOUS THROMBOSIS

The risk of systemic venous thrombosis in children is much lower than it is in adults. Most episodes of VTE in children occur in association with risk factors such as cancer, trauma/surgery, congenital heart disease, and systemic lupus erythematosus. Over 50% of these venous thrombi complicate CVL and occur in arm veins; the majority of the rest occur in leg veins. One randomized trial compared unfractionated heparin (UFH) plus warfarin with the low-molecular-weight heparin (LMWH) reviparin. The study was terminated prior to completion, at which time the recurrence rate was 5.6% in the reviparin arm and 12.5% in the heparin/warfarin arm (a non-significant trend in favor of LMWH).

RENAL VEIN THROMBOSIS

Renal vein thrombosis is responsible for 10% of VTE in neonates and is the most common cause of non–catheter-related VTE in neonates. Data on the effects of antithrombotic therapy for this condition are sparse.

PREVENTION OF CENTRAL VENOUS LINE THROMBOSIS

The effects of fixed-dose warfarin (1 mg) and of LMWH in preventing central line thrombosis have been compared with no treatment in a number of small clinical trials. The results have been inconsistent. One multicenter trial failed to show a difference in the rate of venographic thrombosis between the LMWH reviparin and a non-treated control.

PRIMARY PROPHYLAXIS IN SPECIAL HIGH-RISK GROUPS

There are a number of operative procedures performed in neonates, such as correction of congenital heart abnormalities, that are associated with an increased risk of thrombosis, but there are no reliable data on the relative efficacy and safety of antithrombotic therapy for such procedures. For children with prosthetic heart valves, recommendations for antithrombotic therapy are based on extrapolation from results of trials in adults.

Primary Prophylaxis for Cardiac Catheterization
In the absence of prophylaxis, cardiac catheterization can be complicated by femoral artery thrombosis. Symptomatic TE events have been reported in up to 40% of children who undergo cardiac catheterization. Aspirin does not reduce the risk of TE complications, but heparin reduces the incidence by more than 75%.

TREATMENT OF FEMORAL ARTERY THROMBOSIS AFTER CARDIAC CATHETERIZATION

Children with established femoral vein thrombosis are usually treated with heparin or thrombolytic therapy. There have been no studies evaluating the efficacy of these agents.

UMBILICAL ARTERY CATHETERS

The umbilical artery is often the site of catheterization in sick newborn children who require blood gas analysis and other monitoring. These neonates can develop thromboembolic complications, including aortic thrombosis. Reliable data on the prevention and treatment of umbilical artery thrombosis are not available.

KAWASAKI'S DISEASE

During the acute stage of Kawasaki's disease, children can develop medium and large vessel arteritis and arterial aneurysms, which can lead to arterial stenosis and thrombosis. There is some evidence that IV gamma globulin is effective in preventing this complication. Aspirin in anti-inflammatory doses is also effective.

CEREBRAL VENOUS THROMBOSIS

Cerebral venous thrombosis can occur in neonates and in children. The role of anticoagulants in neonates is controversial, whereas anticoagulants are considered to be appropriate in children, provided there is no intracranial bleeding.

ARTERIAL ISCHEMIC STROKE

Arterial ischemic stroke can occur in neonates and in children. The role of antithrombotic therapy is uncertain, but it is recommended in children with arterial ischemic stroke.

PURPURA FULMINANS

This disorder occurs in homozygous protein C deficiency and, less frequently, in homozygous protein S deficiency. Patients are treated acutely with replacement therapy and long-term with replacement therapy and warfarin.

RECOMMENDATIONS

In neonates with VTE (CVL and non–CVL-related)

1. We suggest that CVLs or umbilical vein catheters (UVCs) associated with confirmed thrombosis be removed, if possible, after 3 to 5 days of anticoagulation **(Grade 2C)**.
2. We suggest either initial anticoagulation, or supportive care with radiologic monitoring **(Grade 2C)**; however, we recommend subsequent anticoagulation if extension of the thrombosis occurs during supportive care **(Grade 1B)**.
3. We suggest anticoagulation should be with either: (1) LMWH given twice daily and adjusted to achieve an anti-factor Xa level of 0.5 to 1.0 U/mL: or (2) UFH for 3 to 5 days adjusted to achieve an anti-factor Xa of 0.35 to 0.7 U/mL or a corresponding activated partial

thromboplastin time (APTT) range, followed by LMWH. We suggest a total duration of anticoagulation of between 6 weeks and 3 months **(Grade 2C)**.

4. We suggest that, if either a CVL or a UVC is still in place on completion of therapeutic anticoagulation, a prophylactic dose of LMWH be given to prevent recurrent VTE until such time as the CVL or UVC is removed **(Grade 2C)**.

5. We recommend against thrombolytic therapy for neonatal VTE unless major vessel occlusion is causing critical compromise of organs or limbs **(Grade 1B)**.

6. We suggest that, if thrombolysis is required, the clinician use tissue plasminogen activator (t-PA) and supplement with plasminogen (fresh frozen plasma) prior to commencing therapy **(Grade 2C)**.

Children with DVT

1. We recommend anticoagulant therapy with either UFH or LMWH **(Grade 1B)**.

2. We recommend initial treatment with UFH or LMWH for at least 5 to 10 days **(Grade 1B)**. For patients in whom clinicians will subsequently prescribe a vitamin K antagonist (VKA), we recommend beginning oral therapy as early as day 1 and discontinuing UFH/LMWH on day 6 (later than day 6 if the INR has not exceeded 2.0) **(Grade 1B)**. After the initial 5- to 10-day treatment period, we suggest LMWH rather than VKA therapy if therapeutic levels are difficult to maintain on VKA therapy or if VKA therapy is challenging for the child and family **(Grade 2C)**.

3. We suggest children with idiopathic TE receive anticoagulant therapy for at least 6 months, using VKAs to achieve a target INR of 2.5 (INR range: 2.0 to 3.0) or, alternatively, using LMWH to maintain an anti-factor Xa level of 0.5 to 1.0 U/mL **(Grade 2C)**.

4. In children with secondary thrombosis in whom the risk factor has resolved, we suggest anticoagulant therapy be administered for at least 3 months using VKAs to achieve a target INR of 2.5 (INR range: 2.0 to 3.0) or, alternatively, using LMWH to maintain an anti-factor Xa level of 0.5 to 1.0 U/mL **(Grade 2C)**.

5. In children who have ongoing, but potentially reversible risk factors, such as active nephrotic syndrome or ongoing L-asparaginase therapy, we suggest continuing anticoagulant therapy in either therapeutic or prophylactic doses until the risk factor has resolved **(Grade 2C)**.

6. For children with recurrent idiopathic thrombosis, we recommend indefinite treatment with VKAs to achieve a target INR of 2.5 (INR range: 2.0 to 3.0) **(Grade 1A)**.

Remark: For some patients, long-term LMWH may be preferable; however, there is little or no data about the safety of long-term LMWH in children.

7. For children with recurrent secondary TEs with an existing reversible risk factor for thrombosis, we suggest anticoagulation until the removal of the precipitating factor, but for a minimum of 3 months **(Grade 2C)**.

8. If a CVL is no longer required, or is nonfunctioning, we recommend it be removed **(Grade 1B)**. We suggest at least 3 to 5 days of anticoagulation therapy prior to its removal **(Grade 2C)**. If CVL access is required and the CVL is still functioning, we suggest that the CVL remain in situ and the patient be anticoagulated **(Grade 2C)**.

9. For children with a first CVL-related DVT, we suggest initial management as for secondary TE as previously described. We suggest that, after the initial 3 months of therapy, prophylactic doses of VKAs (INR range: 1.5 to 1.9) or LMWH (anti-factor Xa level range: 0.1 to 0.3) be given until the CVL is removed **(Grade 2C)**. If recurrent thrombosis occurs while the patient is receiving prophylactic therapy, we suggest continuing therapeutic doses until the CVL is removed (but for at least 3 months) **(Grade 2C)**.

10. In children with DVT, we suggest that thrombolysis therapy not be used routinely **(Grade 2C)**. If thrombolysis is used, in the presence of physiologic or pathologic deficiencies of plasminogen, we suggest supplementation with plasminogen **(Grade 2C)**.

11. If life-threatening VTE is present, we suggest thrombectomy **(Grade 2C)**.

12. We suggest, following thrombectomy, anticoagulant therapy be initiated **(Grade 2C)**.

13. In children > 10 kg body weight with lower-extremity DVT and a contraindication to anticoagulation, we suggest placement of a temporary inferior vena-caval (IVC) filter **(Grade 2C)**.

14. We suggest temporary IVC filters be removed as soon as possible if thrombosis is not present in the basket of the filter and when the risk of anticoagulation decreases **(Grade 2C)**.

15. In children who receive an IVC filter, we recommend appropriate anticoagulation for DVT (see above) as soon as the contraindication to anticoagulation is resolved **(Grade 1B)**.

16. In children with cancer, we suggest that management of VTE follow the general recommendations for management of DVT in children. We suggest the use of LMWH in the treatment of VTE for a minimum of 3 months until the precipitating factor has resolved (eg, use of L-asparaginase) **(Grade 2C)**.

Remark: The presence of cancer, the need for surgery, chemotherapy, or other treatments may modify the risk-benefit ratio for treatment of DVT, and clinicians should consider these factors on an individual basis.

17. We suggest clinicians not use primary antithrombotic prophylaxis in children with cancer and central venous access devices **(Grade 2C)**.

18. For children with VTE, in the setting of APLA, we suggest management as per general recommendations for VTE management in children.
    Remark: Depending on the age of the patient, it may be more appropriate to follow adult guidelines for management of VTE in the setting of APLA.

19. For neonates or children with unilateral renal vein thrombosis (RVT) in the absence of renal impairment or extension into the IVC, we suggest supportive care with monitoring of the RVT for extension or anticoagulation with UFH/LMWH or LMWH in therapeutic doses; we suggest continuation for 3 months **(Grade 2C)**.

20. For unilateral RVT that extends into the IVC, we suggest anticoagulation with UFH/LMWH or LMWH for 3 months **(Grade 2C)**.

21. For bilateral RVT with various degrees of renal failure, we suggest anticoagulation with UFH and initial thrombolytic therapy with t-PA, followed by anticoagulation with UFH/LMWH **(Grade 2C)**.
    Remark: LMWH therapy requires careful monitoring in the presence of significant renal impairment.

22. In children with CVLs, we recommend against the use of routine systemic thromboprophylaxis **(Grade 1B)**.

23. In children receiving long-term home total parenteral nutrition, we suggest thromboprophylaxis with VKAs with a target INR of 2.5 (2.0 to 3.0) **(Grade 2C)**.

24. For blocked CVLs, we suggest t-PA or recombinant urokinase to restore patency **(Grade 2C)**. If, 30 minutes following local thrombolytic instillation, CVL patency is not restored, we suggest a second dose be administered. If the CVL remains blocked following 2 doses of local thrombolytic agent, we suggest investigations to rule out a CVL-related thrombosis be initiated **(Grade 2C)**.

25. For pediatric patients having modified Blalock-Taussig shunt (MBTS), we suggest intraoperative therapy with UFH followed by either aspirin (1 to 5 mg/kg/d) or no further antithrombotic therapy, instead of prolonged LMWH or VKAs **(Grade 2C)**.

26. For patients who underwent the Norwood procedure, we suggest UFH immediately after the procedure, with or without ongoing antiplatelet therapy **(Grade 2C)**.

27. In patients who have bilateral cavopulmonary shunts (BCPS), we suggest postoperative UFH **(Grade 2C)**.

28. For children after Fontan surgery, we recommend aspirin (1 to 5 mg/kg/d) or therapeutic UFH followed by VKAs to achieve a target INR of 2.5 (range: 2.0 to 3.0) **(Grade 1B)**.
Remark: The optimal duration of therapy is unknown, as is whether or not patients with fenestrations require more intensive therapy until fenestration closure.

29. For children having endovascular stents inserted, we suggest administration of UFH perioperatively **(Grade 2C)**.

30. We suggest that pediatric patients with cardiomyopathy receive VKAs to achieve a target INR of 2.5 (range: 2.0 to 3.0) no later than their activation on a cardiac transplant waiting list **(Grade 2C)**.

31. In children with primary pulmonary hypertension, we suggest anticoagulation with VKAs commencing when other medical therapy is commenced **(Grade 2C)**.

32. For children with biologic prosthetic heart valves, we recommend that clinicians follow the relevant recommendations from the adult population.

33. For children with mechanical prosthetic heart valves, we recommend that clinicians follow the relevant recommendations from the adult population with respect to the intensity of anticoagulation therapy.

34. For children with mechanical prosthetic heart valves who have experienced thrombotic events while on therapeutic antithrombotic therapy, or in patients in whom there is a contraindication to full-dose VKAs, we suggest adding aspirin therapy **(Grade 2C)**.

35. Following ventricular assist device (VAD) placement, in the absence of bleeding, we suggest administration of UFH targeted to an anti-factor Xa of 0.35 to 0.7 U/mL **(Grade 2C)**. We suggest starting UFH between 8 and 48 hours following implantation **(Grade 2C)**.

36. We suggest antiplatelet therapy (either aspirin at 1 to 5 mg/kg/d and/or dipyridamole 3 to 10 mg/kg/d) to commence within 72 hours of VAD placement **(Grade 2C)**.

37. We suggest that, once clinically stable, pediatric patients be weaned from UFH to either LMWH (target anti-factor Xa 0.5 to 1.0 U/mL) or VKA (target INR: 3.0 range: 2.5 to 3.5) until transplanted or weaned from VAD **(Grade 2C)**.

38. For neonates and children requiring cardiac catheterization (CC) via an artery, we recommend administration of IV UFH prophylaxis **(Grade 1A)**.

39. We recommend the use of UFH doses of 100 to 150 U/kg as a bolus **(Grade 1B)**. We suggest further doses of UFH rather than no further therapy in prolonged procedures **(Grade 2B)**.

40. We recommend against the use of aspirin therapy for prophylaxis for CC **(Grade 1B)**.

41. For pediatric patients with a femoral artery thrombosis, we recommend therapeutic doses of intravenous UFH **(Grade 1B)**. We suggest treatment for at least 5 to 7 days **(Grade 2C)**.
42. We recommend administration of thrombolytic therapy for pediatric patients with limb-threatening or organ-threatening (via proximal extension) femoral artery thrombosis who fail to respond to initial UFH therapy and who have no known contraindications **(Grade 1B)**.
43. For children with femoral artery thrombosis, we suggest surgical intervention when there is a contraindication to thrombolytic therapy and organ or limb death is imminent **(Grade 2C)**.
44. We suggest, for children in whom thrombolysis or surgery is not required, conversion to LMWH to complete 5 to 7 days of treatment **(Grade 2C)**.
45. For pediatric patients with peripheral arterial catheters in situ, we recommend UFH through the catheter, preferably by continuous infusion (5 U/mL at 1 mL/h) **(Grade 1A)**.
46. For children with a peripheral arterial catheter-related TE, we suggest immediate removal of the catheter **(Grade 1B)**. We suggest UFH anticoagulation with or without thrombolysis, or surgical thrombectomy **(Grade 2C)**.
47. To maintain umbilical artery catheter (UAC) patency, we suggest prophylaxis with a low-dose UFH infusion via the UAC (heparin concentration of 0.25 to 1 U/mL) **(Grade 2A)**.
48. For neonates with UAC-related thrombosis, we suggest therapy with UFH or LMWH for at least 10 days **(Grade 2C)**.
49. For neonates with UAC-related thrombosis, we recommend UAC removal **(Grade 1B)**.
50. For neonates with UAC-related thrombosis with potentially life-, limb-, or organ-threatening symptoms, we suggest thrombolysis with t-Pa. When thrombolysis is contraindicated, we suggest surgical thrombectomy **(Grade 2C)**.
51. We suggest UAC placement in a high, rather than a low, position **(Grade 2B)**.

Neonatal Aortic Thrombosis—Spontaneous

1. In patients undergoing hemodialysis, we suggest against routine use of VKAs or LMWH for prevention of thrombosis related to central venous lines or fistulas. **(Grade 2C)**.
2. We suggest the use of UFH or LMWH in hemodialysis **(Grade 2C)**.
3. In children with Kawasaki's disease, we recommend aspirin in high doses (80 to 100 mg/kg/d during the acute phase, for up to 14 days) as

an anti-inflammatory agent, then in lower doses (1 to 5 mg/kg/d for 6 to 8 weeks) as an antiplatelet agent **(Grade 1B)**.

4. In children with Kawasaki's disease, we suggest against concomitant use of ibuprofen or other non-steroidal anti-inflammatory drugs during aspirin therapy **(Grade 2C)**.

5. In children with Kawasaki's disease, we recommend IV gamma globulin (2 g/kg, single dose) within 10 days of the onset of symptoms **(Grade 1A)**.

6. In children with giant coronary aneurysms following Kawasaki's disease, we suggest warfarin (target INR: 2.5; INR range: 2.0 to 3.0) in addition to therapy with low-dose aspirin be given as primary thromboprophylaxis **(Grade 2C)**.

7. For neonates with cerebral sinovenous thrombosis (CSVT) without significant intracranial hemorrhage, we suggest anticoagulation, initially with UFH or LMWH and, subsequently, with LMWH or VKA for a minimum of 6 weeks, and no longer than 3 months **(Grade 2C)**.

8. For children with CSVT with significant hemorrhage, we suggest radiologic monitoring of the thrombosis at 5 to 7 days and anticoagulation if thrombus propagation is noted **(Grade 2C)**.

9. For children with CSVT without significant intracranial hemorrhage, we recommend anticoagulation, initially with UFH or LMWH, and subsequently, with LMWH or VKA for a minimum of 3 months relative to no anticoagulation **(Grade 1B)**.

10. If, after 3 months of therapy, there is incomplete radiologic recanalization of CSVT (or ongoing symptoms), we suggest administration of a further 3 months of anticoagulation **(Grade 2C)**.

11. For children with CSVT with significant hemorrhage, we suggest radiologic monitoring of the thrombosis at 5 to 7 days. If thrombus propagation is noted at that time, we suggest anticoagulation **(Grade 2C)**.

12. We suggest children with CSVT, in the context of a potentially recurrent risk factors (for example nephrotic syndrome, L-asparaginase therapy) should receive prophylactic anticoagulation at times of risk-factor recurrence **(Grade 2C)**.

13. We suggest thrombolysis thrombectomy or surgical decompression only in children with severe CSVT in whom there is no improvement with initial UFH therapy **(Grade 2C)**.

14. In the absence of a documented ongoing cardioembolic source, we recommend against anticoagulation or aspirin therapy for neonates with a first arterial ischemic stroke (AIS) **(Grade 1B)**.

15. In neonates with recurrent AIS, we suggest anticoagulant or aspirin therapy **(Grade 2C)**.

16. For children with non–sickle-cell-disease-related acute AIS, we recommend UFH or LMWH or aspirin (1 to 5 mg/kg/d) as initial therapy until dissection and embolic causes have been excluded **(Grade 1B)**.

17. We recommend, once dissection and cardioembolic causes are excluded, daily aspirin prophylaxis (1 to 5 mg/kg/d) for a minimum of 2 years **(Grade 1B)**.

18. We suggest, for AIS secondary to dissection or cardioembolic causes, anticoagulant therapy with LMWH or VKAs for at least 6 weeks, with ongoing treatment dependent on radiologic assessment **(Grade 2C)**.

19. We recommend against the use of thrombolysis (t-PA) for AIS in children, outside of specific research protocols **(Grade 1B)**.

20. We recommend, for children with sickle-cell disease and AIS, IV hydration and exchange transfusion to reduce sickle hemoglobin levels to at least < 30% of total hemoglobin **(Grade 1B)**.

21. For children with sickle cell disease and AIS, after initial exchange transfusion, we recommend a chronic transfusion program **(Grade 1B)**.

22. In children with sickle-cell anemia who have transcranial Doppler velocities > 200 cm/s on screening, we recommend regular blood transfusion, which should be continued indefinitely **(Grade 1B)**.

23. We recommend that children with moyamoya disease be referred to an appropriate center for consideration of revascularization **(Grade 1B)**.

24. For children receiving aspirin who have recurrent AIS or transient ischemic attacks, we suggest changing to clopidogrel or anticoagulant (LMWH or VKA) therapy **(Grade 2C)**.

25. For neonates with homozygous protein C deficiency, we recommend administration of either 10 to 20 mL/kg of fresh frozen plasma every 12 hours, or protein C concentrate, when available, at 20 to 60 U/kg until the clinical lesions resolve **(Grade 1B)**.

26. We suggest long-term treatment with vitamin K antagonists **(Grade 2C)**, LMWH **(Grade 2C)**, protein C replacement **(Grade 1B)**, or liver transplantation **(Grade 2C)**.

CHAPTERS AND AUTHORS – ACCP EVIDENCE-BASED CLINICAL PRACTICE GUIDELINES (EIGHTH EDITION):

Antithrombotic and Thrombolytic Therapy – *Jack Hirsh; Gregory W. Albers; Gordon H. Guyatt; Robert A. Harrington; Holger J Schünemann*

Methodology for Antithrombotic and Thrombolytic Therapy Guideline Development – *Holger Schunemann; Deborah J. Cook; Gordon H. Guyatt*

Grades of Recommendation for Antithrombotic Agents – *Gordon Guyatt; Holger J. Schünemann; Deborah J. Cook; Roman Jaeschke; Stephen G. Pauker*

Strategies for Incorporating Resource Allocation and Economic Considerations – *Daniel Mark, David Matchar*

Parenteral Anticoagulants – *Jack Hirsh ; Kenneth A. Bauer; Maria B. Donati; Michael Gould; Meyer M. Samama; Jeffrey I. Weitz*

The Pharmacology and Management of the Vitamin K Antagonists – *Jack Ansell; Jack Hirsh; Alan Jacobson; Elaine Hylek; Mark Crowther; Gualtiero Palareti*

Antiplatelet Drugs – *Carlo Patrono; Jack Hirsh; Gerald Roth; Colin Baigent*

New Antithrombotic Drugs – *Jeffrey Weitz; Jack Hirsh; Meyer M. Samama*

Hemorrhagic Complications of Anticoagulant and Thrombolytic Treatment – *Sam Schulman; Mark N. Levine; Rebecca J. Beyth; Clive Kearon*

The Perioperative Management of Antithrombotic Therapy – *Jack Ansell, James Douketis; Andrew S. Dunn; Amir K. Jaffer; Richard C. Becker; Alex C. Spyropoulos; Peter B. Berger*

Treatment and Prevention of Heparin-Induced Thrombocytopenia – *Theodore Warkentin ; Andreas Greinacher; A. Michael Lincoff; Andreas Koste*

Prevention of Venous Thromboembolism – *William Geerts ; David Bergqvist; Clifford W. Colwell; John A. Heit; Michael R. Lassen; Charles M. Samama; Graham F. Pineo*

Antithrombotic Therapy for Venous Thromboembolic Disease – *Clive Kearon; Giancarlo Agnelli; Samuel Goldhaber; Gary E. Raskob; Anthony J. Comerota; Susan R. Kahn*

Antithrombotic Therapy in Atrial Fibrillation – *Daniel Singer; Gregory W. Albers; James E. Dalen; Margaret C. Fang; Alan S. Go; Jonathan L. Halperin; Warren J. Manning; Gregory Y. H. Lip*

Valvular and Structural Heart Disease – *Deeb Salem; Patrick T. O'Gara; Stephen G. Pauker; Christopher Madias*

INDEX

Desmoteplase, 34
for acute ischemic stroke, 34
Diclofenac
for infusion thrombophlebitis, 78
Dipyridamole, 20–21
absorption, 21
for arterial thrombosis prevention and
treatment, 17
for cerebral ischemic events, 102
for NSTE ACS, 104
for stroke prevention, 97–98
VAD placement, 146
Direct factor Xa inhibitors, 30
Direct thrombin inhibitors (DTI), 8–10
for acute STEMI, 119
bleeding risk, 36
management of, 49
monitoring of, 10
for NSTE, 106–107
recommendations, 10
for STEMI, 114
Drotrecogin alfa (activated), 32
DTI. See Direct thrombin inhibitors (DTI)
Dual antiplatelet therapy, 124
DU-176b, 32
Duplex ultrasound (DUS) screening, 61
DUS. See Duplex ultrasound (DUS) screening
DVT. See Deep vein thrombosis (DVT)
DX9065a, 30

E
E5555, 27
EAFT. See European Atrial Fibrillation Trial
(EAFT)
Elastic stockings
for postthrombotic syndrome of arm, 80
preventing PTS, 73–74
for PTS without venous leg ulcers, 74
Elective cardioversion
of AF
anticoagulation for, 86
IV UFH for, 86
anticoagulation for, 83
Elective hip replacement
VTE, 59

Elective hip surgery
fondaparinux for, 53
LMWH for, 53
oral anticoagulants for, 53
Elective knee replacement
VTE, 59–60
Elective spine surgery
VTE, 61
Embolic stroke
aortic atheromata causing, 99
causes of, 99
Emergency cardioversion
of atrial fibrillation, 84
Endothelial-derived proteins, 4
Endovascular stents
children
Grade 2C, 146
UFH, 146
Enoxaparin
vs. rivaroxaban, 31
Enoxaparin and Thrombolysis Reperfusion
for Acute Myocardial
Infarction Treatment,
Thrombolysis in
Myocardial Infarction-
Study 25 (ExTRACT-
TIMI 25) trial, 113
Environmental factors
VKA, 12–13
EPIC. See Evaluation of c7E3 to Prevent
Ischemic Complica-
tions (EPIC) trial
EPILOG. See Evaluation in PTCA to
Improve Long-Term
Outcome with Abcix-
imab GP IIb/IIIa
Blockade (EPILOG)
trial
EPISTENT. See Evaluation of Platelet
IIb/IIIa Inhibitor for
Stenting Trial (EPIS-
TENT)
Eptifibatide, 24
for arterial thrombosis prevention and
treatment, 17
for NSTE ACS, 104, 105, 108

Mechanical heart valve replacement
VKA, 122
Mechanical prosthetic valves, 89–90
children, 146
aspirin therapy, 146
Grade 2C, 146
VKA, 146
in pregnancy
anticoagulant management of, 139
Grade 1C, 139
Grade 2C, 139
LMWH, 139
UFH, 139
Mechanical valve
bileaflet, 92
Medical conditions, 53–54
VTE risk factors, 64
Medtronic-Hall tilting disc mechanical
valves, 89, 92
MI. *See* Myocardial infarction (MI)
Micronized purified flavonoid fraction
for venous leg ulcers, 74
Mitral annular calcification (MAC), 88, 92
aspirin for, 92
Mitral regurgitation, 87–88
Mitral stenosis, 87–88
percutaneous balloon mitral valvulo-
plasty for, 88
TEE for, 88
Mitral valve prolapse (MVP), 88, 91
Grade 1B, 91
with ischemic stroke, 99
Moderate-quality evidence, 2
Modified Blalock-Taussig shunt (MBTS)
Grade 2C, 145
UFH, 145
Monitoring antithrombotic effect, 10
Moyamoya disease
children
Grade 1B, 148
revascularization, 148
MVP. *See* Mitral valve prolapse (MVP)
Myocardial infarction (MI), 7
aspirin, 125
aspirin for, 19–20
Grade 2A, 125

VKA for, 121, 125
warfarin INR for, 121

N
Nadroparin, 52
NAPc2, 28
Natural pentasaccharide, 6
NBTE. *See* Nonbacterial thrombotic endo-
carditis (NBTE)
Neonates
antithrombotic therapy, 140–149
aortic thrombosis, 147–149
CC
aspirin therapy, 146
Grade 1A, 146
Grade 1B, 146
IV UFH, 146
CSVT
Grade 1B, 148
Grade 2C, 148
LMWH, 148
UFH, 148
VKA, 148
homozygous protein C deficiency, 148
Grade 1B, 148
Grade 2C, 148
LMWH, 148
plasma, 148
protein C, 148
RVT, 145
UAC
Grade 2C, 147
LMWH, 147
UFH, 147
umbilical artery catheters, 141
VTE, 142–143
Grade 1B, 142, 143
Grade 2C, 142
LMWH, 142–143
VTE anticoagulation, 142
Neuraxial anesthesia analgesia
antithrombotic therapy, 55
Neurosurgery
VTE, 62
Newborn. *See* Neonates
Nonbacterial thrombotic endocarditis
(NBTE), 90–95

Subcutaneous (SC) injection, 4
Subcutaneous (SC) intravenous (IV) unfrac-
   tionated heparin (UFH)
 for acute leg DVT, 70
 for DVT, 66, 67, 71
 for PE, 74
Subcutaneous (SC) low-molecular-weight
   heparin (LMWH),
   40, 41
 for acute leg DVT, 70
 for PE, 74
Sulodexide
 for venous leg ulcers, 74
Superficial thrombophlebitis, 70
 LMWH for, 70
 UFH for, 70
Superficial vein thrombosis
 Grade 1B, 78
 Grade 2B, 78
 Grade 2C, 78
 LMWH for, 78
 NSAID for, 78
 treatment of, 78
 UFH for, 78
 VKA, 78
Superior vena caval filter insertion
 for UEDVT, 79
Superior Yield of the New Strategy of
   Enoxaparin, Revascu-
   larization and Glyco-
   protein IIb/IIIa
   Inhibitors (SYN-
   ERGY) trial, 106
Surgical thrombectomy
 for UEDVT, 79
SYNERGY. *See* Superior Yield of the New
   Strategy of Enoxa-
   parin, Revasculariza-
   tion and Glycoprotein
   IIb/IIIa Inhibitors
   (SYNERGY) trial
Systemic thrombolytic therapy
 for acute DVT, 72
 for DVT, 67
Systemic venous thrombosis
 children, 140

 LMWH, 140
 reviparin, 140
 UFH, 140
 warfarin, 140

T
TARGET. *See* Tirofiban and Reopro Give
   Similar Efficacy Out-
   comes (TARGET)
   study
TEE. *See* Transesophageal echocardiography
   (TEE)
Tenecteplase
 for acute STEMI, 119
 comparison of, 110
Therapeutic-dose unfractionated heparin
 platelet count monitoring of patients
   receiving, 46–47
Thienopyridines, 21–23, 26
 for NSTE ACS, 104
 PCI, 126
Thoracic surgery
 VTE, 58
THR. *See* Total hip replacement (THR)
Thrombectomy
 VTE, 144
Thrombin inhibitors, 32–33
Thrombolysis, 129
 Grade 2C, 143
 t-PA, 143
Thrombolysis in Myocardial Infarction 28
   (TIMI 28), 120
Thrombolytic therapy
 bleeding risk, 36
 DVT children, 144
 femoral artery thrombosis after cardiac
   catheterization, 141
 hemorrhagic complications of, 35–37
 for ischemic stroke, 96–97
 for PE, 69, 76
 for UEDVT, 79
Thrombophilia, 133–139
 aspirin, 138
 Grade 1A, 138
 Grade 1B, 138
 LMWH, 138

LMWH, 147
UFH, 147
UFH, 147
Umbilical vein catheters (UVC), 142
Unexplained cerebral ischemia
    DVT, 89
Unfractionated heparin (UFH), 3, 5, 25, 41.
                    See also Intravenous
                        unfractionated heparin
    acute VTE, 136
    atherosclerotic PAD, 128
    BCPS, 145
    cardiopulmonary bypass surgery, 46
    for cerebral venous sinus thrombosis, 103
    chronic AF, 39
    CSVT neonates, 148
    for DVT, 66
    DVT children, 143
    endovascular stents children, 146
    femoral artery thrombosis children, 147
    Fontan surgery children, 146
    hemorrhagic complications of, 35
    MBTS, 145
    mechanical prosthetic valves in preg-
                        nancy, 139
    neonatal CSVT, 148
    neonatal UAC, 147
    Norwood procedure, 145
    for NSTE, 105, 106–107
    for NSTE ACS, 108
    for PE, 74
    platelet count monitoring, 47
    during pregnancy, 134
    for prophylaxis, 52
    prosthetic heart valves, 38–39
    recurrent VTE in pregnancy women, 137
    RVT, 145
    for STEMI, 112, 117
    for superficial thrombophlebitis, 70
    for superficial vein thrombosis, 78
    systemic venous thrombosis, 140
    therapeutic-dose
        platelet count monitoring of patients
                        receiving, 46–47
    timing decisions with, 38
    UAC, 147

VAD, 146
VTE, 39
Unstable angina
    LMWH for, 6
Upper extremity deep vein thrombosis
                    (UEDVT), 70–80
    anticoagulants for, 79
    catheter extraction for, 79
    Grade 1C, 79
    Grade 2C, 79
    IV UFH for, 79
    LMWH for, 79
    recommendations for, 70–80
    staged approach of lysis for, 79
    stent placement for, 79
    superior vena caval filter insertion for, 79
    surgical thrombectomy for, 79
    thrombolytic therapy for, 79
    transluminal angioplasty for, 79
Urgent surgical procedures, 40
    management of, 40
    recommendations for, 40–44
Urologic surgery
    VTE, 57–58
UVC. *See* Umbilical vein catheters (UVC)

V
VAD. *See* Ventricular assist device (VAD)
                        placement
Valvular heart disease, 87–95
    atrial fibrillation, 83, 85
Variable international normalized ratio
    management of, 17
Vascular surgery
    with HIT history, 50
    intravenous UFH, 132
    risk categories, 52
    VTE, 56
Vena cava filters
    for CTPH, 78
    for DVT, 72
    for PE, 76
Venous foot pump (VFP)
    reducing venous stasis, 52
Venous leg ulcers
    Grade 2B, 74